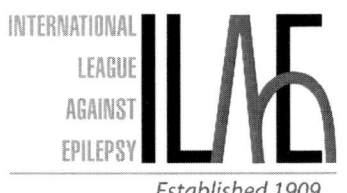
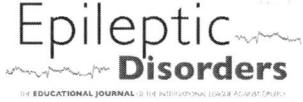

Volume 18, May 2016 • Supplement I

Psychiatric and Behavioural Disorders in Children with Epilepsy

Report of the Child Neuropsychiatry Taskforce, Neuropsychobiology Commission, International League Against Epilepsy

Guest Editor:
Frank MC Besag

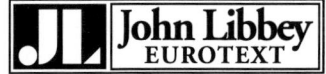

Members of the immediate past Child Neuropsychiatry Taskforce
Albert Aldenkamp (The Netherlands)
Frank Besag (UK, Chairperson)
Rochelle Caplan (USA)
David Dunn (USA)
Giuseppe Gobbi (Italy)
Matti Sillanpää (Finland)

Acknowledgements
The task force is grateful for the assistance of Roberto Tuchman with the paper on autism and both Helen Cross and Mary Lou Smith with the paper on surgery. The extensive technical assistance of Tom Hawking and Gariba Awudu is also very gratefully acknowledged. We thank Andres Kanner and Marco Mula for their constant support and Kousuke Kanemoto for his very kind encouragement.

Potential conflicts of interest and financial support

Name	Any conflicts of interest	Any financial support
Albert Aldenkamp	No	No
Frank Besag	No	No
Rochelle Caplan	No	No
David W. Dunn	No	Receives grant support from Eli Lilly through the Indiana University School of Medicine
Giuseppe Gobbi	No	No
Matti Sillanpää	No	No

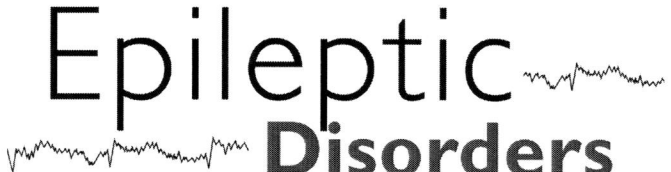

The Educational Journal of the International League Against Epilepsy
HTTP://WWW.EPILEPTICDISORDERS.COM

EDITOR-IN-CHIEF
Alexis A. Arzimanoglou
Director, Epilepsy, Sleep and Pediatric Neurophysiology Dpt.
University Hospitals of Lyon, France
Consultant, Hospital San Juan de Dios, Barcelona, Spain

FOUNDING EDITOR
Jean Aicardi
Paris, France

ASSOCIATE EDITORS

Ingmar Blümcke
Erlangen, Germany

François Dubeau
Montreal, Canada

Michael Duchowny
Miami, USA

Aristea Galanopoulou
New York, USA

Alexander Hammers
Lyon, France

Yushi Inoue
Shizuoka, Japan

Philippe Kahane
Grenoble, France

Michael Kerr
Cardiff, UK

Silvia Kochen
Buenos Aires, Argentina

Carla Marini
Florence, Italy

Doug Nordli
Chicago, USA

Graeme Sills
Liverpool, UK

Pierre Thomas
Nice, France

Torbjorn Tomson
Stockholm, Sweden

Sarah Wilson
Melbourne, Australia

DEPUTY EDITORS for *EPILEPSIA*

Gary W. Mathern
Los Angeles, USA

Astrid Nehlig
Paris, France

EDITORIAL BOARD

Andreas Alexopoulos
Cleveland, USA

Fred Andermann
Montreal, Canada

Nadia Bahi-Buisson
Paris, France

Eduardo Baragan
Mexico City, Mexico

Fabrice Bartolomei
Marseille, France

Thomas Bast
Kork, Germany

Selim Benbadis
Tampa, USA

Frank Besag
Bedford, UK

Paul Boon
Gent, Belgium

Patricia Braga
Montevideo, Uruguay

Kees Braun
Utrecht, The Netherlands

Peter Camfield
Halifax, Canada

Giuseppe Capovilla
Mantova, Italy

Mar Carreno
Barcelona, Spain

Jaime Carrizosa
Colombia, Colombia

Francine Chassoux
Paris, France

Dana Craiu
Bucharest, Romania

Antoine Depaulis
Grenoble, France

Petia Dimova
Sofia, Bulgaria

Christian Elger
Bonn, Germany

Pete Engel
Los Angeles, USA

Andras Fogarasi
Budapest, Hungary

Antonio Gil-Nagel
Madrid, Spain

Giuseppe Gobbi
Bologna, Italy

Gregory Holmes
Vermont, USA

Hans Holthausen
Vogtareuth, Germany

Angelina Kakooza
Kampala, Uganda

Andres Kanner
Miami, USA

Peter Kaplan
Baltimore, USA

Eric Kossof
Baltimore, USA

Michalis Koutroumanidis
London, UK

Guenter Kraemer
Zürich, Switzerland

Pavel Krsek
Prague, Czech Republic

Lieven Lagae
Leuven, Belgium

Shih-Hui Lim
Singapore

Hans Lüders
Cleveland, USA

Andrew L. Lux
Bristol, UK

Marco Medina
Tegucigalpa, Honduras

Mohamad Mikati
Durham, USA

Cigdem Ozkara
Istanbul, Turkey

Guido Rubboli
Dianalund, Denmark

Bertil Rydenhag
Goteborg, Sweden

Ingrid Scheffer
Melbourne, Australia

Margitta Seeck
Geneva, Switzerland

Sanjay Sisodiya
London, UK

Michael Sperling
Philadelphia, USA

Roberto Spreafico
Milano, Italy

John Stephenson
Glasgow, Scotland

Pierre Szepetowski
Marseille, France

CT Tan
Kuala Lumpur, Malaysia

Laura Tassi
Milano, Italy

Anna Maria Vezzani
Milano, Italy

Karen S. Wilcox
Salt Lake City, USA

Jo Wilmshurst
Cape Town, South Africa

Elza Marcia Yacubian
Sao Paolo, Brazil

ILAE MANAGEMENT COMMITTEE

Emilio Perucca, President
Pavia, Italy

Samuel Wiebe
Calgary, Canada

J. Helen Cross
London, UK

Tatsuya Tanaka
Asahikawa, Japan

Solomon Moshé
Bronx, NY, USA

EDITORIAL & PRODUCTION STAFF

MANAGING EDITOR
Oliver Gubbay
epileptic.disorders@gmail.com

PUBLICATIONS DIRECTOR
Gilles Cahn
gilles.cahn@jle.com

DESK EDITOR
Marine Rivière
marine.riviere@jle.com

PRODUCT MANAGER
Jiriane Kouevi
jiriane.kouevi@jle.com

ADVERTISING DIRECTOR
Marie-Christine Lasserre
marie-christine.lasserre@jle.com

ISBN: 978-2-7420-1500-9
ISSN: 1294-9361

Published by
Éditions John Libbey Eurotext
127, avenue de la République, 92120 Montrouge, France
Tel.: +33 (0)1 46 73 06 60
www.jle.com

John Libbey Eurotext
42-46 High Street, Esther, Surrey, KT10 9KY
United Kingdom

© 2016, John Libbey Eurotext. All rights reserved.

Unauthorized duplication contravenes applicable laws.
It is prohibited to reproduce this work or any part of it without the authorization of the publisher or of the Centre Français d'Exploitation du Droit de Copie (CFC), 20, rue des Grands-Augustins, 75006 Paris.

Contents

Preface VII

List of authors IX

Epidemiology of psychiatric/behavioural disorder in children with epilepsy
*Matti Sillanpää, Frank Besag, Albert Aldenkamp, Rochelle Caplan,
David W. Dunn, Giuseppe Gobbi* 1

Epilepsy and ADHD
*Frank Besag, Giuseppe Gobbi, Rochelle Caplan, Matti Sillanpää,
Albert Aldenkamp, David W. Dunn* 9

Epilepsy and autism
*Frank Besag, Albert Aldenkamp, Rochelle Caplan, David W. Dunn,
Giuseppe Gobbi, Matti Sillanpää* 21

Anxiety, depression and childhood epilepsy
*David W. Dunn, Frank Besag, Rochelle Caplan, Albert Aldenkamp,
Giuseppe Gobbi, Matti Sillanpää* 31

Epilepsy and psychosis in children and teenagers
*Frank Besag, Rochelle Caplan, Albert Aldenkamp, David W. Dunn,
Giuseppe Gobbi, Matti Sillanpää* 41

Behavioural and psychiatric disorders associated with epilepsy syndromes
*Frank Besag, Giuseppe Gobbi, Albert Aldenkamp, Rochelle Caplan,
David W. Dunn, Matti Sillanpää* 49

Subtle behavioural and cognitive manifestations of epilepsy
*Frank Besag, Giuseppe Gobbi, Albert Aldenkamp, Rochelle Caplan,
David W. Dunn, Matti Sillanpää* 67

Adverse cognitive and behavioural effects of antiepileptic drugs in children
*Albert Aldenkamp, Frank Besag, Giuseppe Gobbi, Rochelle Caplan,
David W. Dunn, Matti Sillanpää* 75

Behavioural effects of epilepsy surgery
Frank Besag, Rochelle Caplan, Albert Aldenkamp, David W. Dunn, Giuseppe Gobbi, Matti Sillanpää.. 95

When should pharmacotherapy for psychiatric/behavioural disorders in children with epilepsy be prescribed?
Frank Besag, Albert Aldenkamp, Rochelle Caplan, David W. Dunn, Giuseppe Gobbi, Matti Sillanpää.. 107

Report of the ILAE Child Neuropsychiatry Taskforce, Neuropsychobiology Commission, published as an e-supplement in *Epileptic Disorders* (Volume 8, May 2016), educational journal of the International League Against Epilepsy.

Preface

Psychiatric/behavioural problems are common in children with epilepsy, typically occurring in around 35-50% in epidemiological studies. They can affect the quality of life of the children and their families to a major degree. In many cases these problems create more of a challenge than the epilepsy itself. However, there are relatively few high-quality studies in this area.

This collection of papers is intended to represent one step in a long journey towards addressing the lack of information by drawing together the available data on a number of key topics including epidemiology, the relationships between epilepsy and several psychiatric disorders, the role of the epilepsy itself, the effects of antiepileptic drugs and surgery and the place of pharmacotherapy.

Although there is relatively good information on epidemiology there is very little information on the causes of and risk factors for psychiatric disorders in childhood epilepsy that might give insight into early diagnosis and prevention.

Despite the growing amount of research in genetics, the impact on management has been minimal so far. There is also very sparse high-quality randomised controlled trial data on treatment of psychiatric disorders in childhood epilepsy. Furthermore, with a few exceptions, there is a striking lack of neuroimaging studies in this field. These are areas that would benefit from further attention and research.

The information in this report has been put together by the members of the immediate past Child Neuropsychiatry Taskforce of the Neuropsychology Commission of the International League Against Epilepsy, guided by the then chairpersons of the commission: Andres Kanner and Marco Mula. The immediate past Task Force was officially in place from July 2009 to June 2013, although their work has continued since then, in relation to this publication and updating all the papers.

**Frank Besag, Albert Aldenkamp, Rochelle Caplan,
David W. Dunn, Giuseppe Gobbi, Matti Sillanpää**

List of authors

Albert Aldenkamp, Professor Dr., Department of Research and Development, Epilepsy Center Kempenhaeghe, Heeze, The Netherlands; MHENS School of Mental Health & Neuroscience, Maastricht University, Maastricht, The Netherlands

Frank Besag, MB ChB, Professor, Mid Beds Clinic, East London NHS Foundation Trust, Bedford, United Kingdom

Rochelle Caplan, MD, Professor, Semel Institute for Neuroscience and Human Behavior, University of California, Los Angeles, California, USA

David W. Dunn, MD, Professor of Psychiatry and Neurology, Riley Hospital Child and Adolescent Psychiatry Clinics, Indiana University School of Medicine, Indianapolis, Indiana, USA

Giuseppe Gobbi, MD, IRCCS – Institute of Neurological Sciences of Bologna, Child Neurology Unit, Bologna, Italy

Matti Sillanpää, MD PhD, Professor Dr. emer., Senior Research Scientist, Depts. Public Health and Child Neurology, University of Turku, Turku, Finland

Epidemiology of psychiatric/behavioural disorder in children with epilepsy

Matti Sillanpää, Frank Besag, Albert Aldenkamp,
Rochelle Caplan, David W. Dunn, Giuseppe Gobbi

Abstract

Psychiatric/behavioural problems can have a major effect on quality of life. Epidemiological studies in Europe, Scandinavia and the USA have confirmed a high rate of psychiatric disorder in children with epilepsy, typically around 350 to 50%. In children with additional impairment, particularly those with intellectual disability, the rates are even higher, over 50%. Determining the causes of these high rates and deciding on the best strategies, either for prevention or for optimal management, remain major challenges.

Key words: epidemiology, population, psychiatric, behavior

Psychiatric and cognitive problems in children with epilepsy can affect quality of life to a major extent (Hermann et al., 2012; Speechley et al., 2012). Long-term follow-up studies show that childhood-onset epilepsy has a marked impact on adult life (Sillanpää et al., 1998; Shackleton et al., 2003) even when the epilepsy is not complicated by intellectual disability or other neurological impairments (Jalava et al., 1997; Sillanpää et al., 1998; Rantanen et al., 2010; Sillanpää, 2010).

■ Search strategy

In addition to studies already known to the authors, the Medline/PubMed database was searched from inception until the end of March 2015 using the search terms: epilep$ and (child$ or pediat$ or adolescen$) and (behav$ or psychiat$) and (epidemiolog$ or population). Abstracts of likely relevance to the topic were examined to select papers for final detailed review. Reference lists of included papers were searched for any further relevant studies.

■ Epidemiological studies

The best way of obtaining accurate information on the prevalence of behavioural/psychiatric problems in children with epilepsy is to examine data from well-designed, carefully-conducted epidemiological studies on large populations of children. Several epidemiological studies have been published.

The classic UK Isle of Wight study (Rutter et al., 1970), performed over 40 years ago, revealed that the rate of psychiatric disorder in complicated epilepsy (children with "lesions above the brainstem") was 58%. The comparable rates for controls were 7% and in children with physical disability 11%. The prevalence of psychiatric disorder in children with uncomplicated epilepsy was 38%. Uncomplicated epilepsy was associated with specific underachievement in reading in 18% compared with 7% of controls. Similar results were reported by others (Stores, 1978; Long and Moore, 1979). Thirty years later, the reported rates of behavioural difficulties were largely similar (Davies et al., 2003 – see later).

Sillanpää (1992) performed a population-based study of long-term illnesses in the western province of Turku and Pori in Finland. Using stratified cluster sampling of health centres, six of 32 health centres (total population 516,000) were randomly chosen for the study. The number of children aged 4-15 years in the area of the six health centres totalled 21,108. Intensive instruction and continuing guidance was given to the health-centre staff. Any long-term illness (defined as the minimum duration of six months, in accordance with the National Health Service statutes) was found in 532 children. To recognise behavioural disturbance, the WHO classification (1980) was applied. The staff were instructed on several occasions how to apply the WHO criteria for behavioural disturbance and the interpretations were discussed to minimise inter-observer variation. Altogether, 96 children with epilepsy were ascertained. The prevalence of life-time epilepsy was 0.7%; 57% had been in one-year remission at examination. Rates of neuropsychological comorbidities were remarkably high: intellectual disability (IQ < 70) in 31%, specific learning difficulties but an intact global intelligence in 23% and "minimal brain dysfunction" in 10%; the rate of enuresis was also high at 20%.

In a study performed four years after the baseline (Sillanpää, 1987), in children and adolescents then aged 8-19 years, any behavioural disturbance was found in 58% of children with epilepsy in comparison with 76%, 83%, 58%, 53% and 67% among children with cerebral palsy, "minimal brain dysfunction", asthma, diabetes or heart disease, respectively. In matched controls, the corresponding behaviour was found in 11%. The behaviour of children with epilepsy was classified as "less polite" or "rude" in 6%, in comparison with 10%, 12%, 6%, 2% and 7% among children with cerebral palsy, "minimal brain dysfunction", asthma, diabetes or heart disease, respectively. In matched controls, the corresponding behaviour occurred in 1%. Disturbed behaviour occurred often or fairly often in 15% of children with epilepsy compared with 5-17% among other children with the above-mentioned illnesses and with 1% of controls. Using the WHO "International Classification of Impairments, Disabilities, and Handicaps", disabilities and handicaps were significantly higher in children with epilepsy than in matched controls: communication disabilities (28% vs 7%), situational disabilities (31% vs 16%), orientation handicap (11% vs 0.3%) and social integration handicap (12% vs 1%). The rate of any handicap was 21% compared with 1% among controls.

Table 1. Using data from Sillanpää (1986) (see text for details of study)

Condition	Epilepsy	Matched controls	Cerebral palsy	"Minimal brain dysfunction"	Asthma	Diabetes	Heart disease
% Any behavioural disturbance	58	11	76	83	58	53	76
% "Less polite" or "rude"	6	1	10	12	6	2	7
% Disturbed behaviour often or fairly often	15	1	←———— 5-17 ————→				

Behavioural problems are more common in children with uncomplicated epilepsy than in controls (Jalava et al., 1997; Sillanpää et al., 1998; Rantanen et al., 2010; Sillanpää, 2010). That difference seems to exist from the very beginning of epilepsy.

Hoie et al. (2008) carried out an epidemiological study of epilepsy in 6-12 year-old children in Norway. They found a significantly higher prevalence of psychosocial problems: 45% compared with 10% in controls. They also found more executive function problems: 31% compared with 11% in controls.

Davies et al. (2003), in a study based on the 1999 British Child and Adolescent Mental Health Survey, found rates of psychiatric disorder that were remarkably similar to those found in the Isle of Wight study (shown in brackets). The overall rate of psychiatric disorder was 37% (38% for "uncomplicated epilepsy"), with a much higher rate of 56% (58%) in complicated epilepsy, compared with 9% (7%) in controls and 11% in children with diabetes (11% in children with physical disability).

Alfstad et al. (2011) carried out a population-based study in Norwegian children aged 8-13 years, using the Strengths and Difficulties Questionnaire, parent form. Of the 110 children with epilepsy, 38% had psychiatric symptoms compared with 17% of controls ($p < 0.001$). They also found that girls had more emotional problems, whereas boys had more peer-relationship difficulties and features of attention deficit hyperactivity disorder (ADHD). Additional independent risk factors for developing psychiatric disorder in children with epilepsy were low socio-economic status and having other chronic diseases such as asthma or diabetes.

In a study from the USA, Russ et al. (2012), using data from the 2007 National Survey of Children's Health (NSCH), reported on the prevalence of psychiatric disorders in children with epilepsy. This survey was on a total of 91,600 children, from birth to 17 years. It included 977 children who were reported by their parents as having been diagnosed with epilepsy or seizure disorder. Psychiatric disorders were statistically significantly more common in children with a current seizure disorder than in those who had never been diagnosed with such a disorder. The respective figures for specific psychiatric disorders were: ADHD 23% vs 6%, anxiety 17% vs 3%, conduct problems 16% vs 3%, depression

8% vs 2% and autism spectrum disorder 16% vs 1%. All these differences were statistically significant ($p < 0.05$). Developmental delay 51% vs 3% was also significantly more common ($p < 0.05$).

In a community-based study in schools in Sussex, UK, Reilly et al. (2014) reported that 80% of 85 children with active epilepsy had neurobehavioural disorder and/or cognitive impairment. The most common neurobehavioural comorbidities were ADHD (33%), autism spectrum disorder (21%) and developmental coordination disorder (18%). Cognitive impairment (IQ < 85) was diagnosed in 55% and intellectually disability (IQ < 70) in 40%. Using the Autism Spectrum Screening Questionnaire, Reilly et al. (2015) also characterised autism spectrum disorder in more detail and found that autistic features were more common in children with epilepsy regardless of cognitive ability.

■ Prevalence at or before the onset of the epilepsy

It has become increasingly apparent that more children at diagnosis of epilepsy have neuropsychological problems than their peers (Rutter et al., 1970; Bourgeois et al., 1983; McDermott et al., 1995). Several publications, including the original study by Rutter et al. (Rutter et al., 1970; Bourgeois et al., 1983; McDermott et al., 1995), have made it clear that the lower the cognitive ability, the higher the prevalence of psychiatric disorder. For this reason, results on cognitive and psychiatric problems will be reported together. Bourgeois et al. (1983) followed the IQ of children with new-onset epilepsy at baseline (within two weeks from the onset of epilepsy) and then annually. In 72 children, the mean IQ was not significantly different from the siblings except for 11 who had a persistent decrease in IQ. Those children were treated with antiepileptic drugs approaching the toxic range and had an earlier age of onset of epilepsy than the others. Before the initiation of drug therapy, the children with idiopathic epilepsy had a higher IQ, a better attention span and better motor and psychomotor ability than those with symptomatic epilepsy.

Hermann et al. (2006) confirmed the results of Oostrom et al. (2003), in 75 children with new-onset epilepsy. Compared with 63 healthy controls, aged 8-18, a comprehensive neuropsychological test battery revealed mild cognitive impairment in intelligence, language, attention, executive function and psychomotor speed. A structured interview with the parents revealed that many kinds of individualised supportive education had also been given to the children with epilepsy. Additionally, prior to the onset of the epilepsy, children had significantly higher rates of depressive disorder (23%), anxiety disorder (36%) and ADHD (26%) than controls.

Rathouz et al. (2014) examined 69 children with new or recent-onset epilepsy shortly after diagnosis and five to six years later, with regard to intelligence, academic achievement, language, executive function and psychomotor speed, compared with 62 controls. Children with epilepsy performed significantly less well than their controls near the time of diagnosis; these findings persisted virtually unchanged over time, without progressive deterioration or recovery. The observations of Bonilha et al. (2014) on 39 children with new-onset epilepsy, compared with 28 healthy controls, suggested abnormal localized and bilateral hemispheric network organization with localization-related epilepsies and generalized epilepsies, respectively. In particular, children with epilepsy, low intelligence level and poor executive function had a suboptimal topographical structural organization with enhanced network segregation and reduced global integration. The same study group

(Almane et al., 2014) showed that behavioural problems and lower social competence were significantly more common in children with new-onset epilepsy compared with controls, regardless of the type of syndrome.

Hoare (1984) studied possible differences in the prevalence of behavioural problems between new-onset and chronic epilepsy. Based on parental behaviour questionnaires, during the first three months from the onset of epilepsy, problems occurred in 45% compared with 48% in children with chronic epilepsy. In controls, only 10% had behavioural problems.

Dunn et al. (1997), in a study of 42 children, found that those in whom the first seizure was followed by additional seizures were at higher risk of behavioural disturbances than children who had no further seizures.

Fastenau et al. (2009), in a large community-based cohort of 282 children, aged 6-14, with an IQ of 70 or more, reported that 27% of children with a single seizure had neuropsychological problems at or near the onset of the epilepsy. Compared with 147 sibling controls, absence epilepsy, which was associated with a doubling of risk, was almost as strong a risk factor as multiple seizures, antiepileptic drug therapy and symptomatic or cryptogenic seizure aetiology.

Oostrom et al. (2003), in a study of 51 children aged 5-16 years with newly-diagnosed epilepsy (either idiopathic or symptomatic) and 48 healthy classmates as controls, found significantly poorer performance associated with epilepsy. On psychological examination of the children with uncomplicated epilepsy ("epilepsy-only") within 48 hours of the onset and prior to drug therapy, a significantly poorer achievement was found in attention, reaction time, visual memory and behaviour; poorer academic skills were also found in the children with epilepsy but the difference did not quite reach statistical significance ($p = 0.07$).

There is some evidence that neuropsychiatric and neurobehavioural changes are present even before the first epileptic seizure. These changes are to be separated from the brief (typically from a few minutes to a few days) prodromal affective and behavioural disturbances preceding a single seizure or cluster of seizures (Hughes et al., 1993; Bjoernaes, 2001).

Austin et al. (2001) carried out a controlled, prospective, population-based study of 224 children with epilepsy aged 4-14 years and their 135 siblings. Behavioural problems were assessed, based on parental reports, in the six months before the first recognised epileptic seizure. Parents rated the behavioural changes on the Child Behaviour Checklist. Total Behaviour Problem scores and Internalizing Problems scores were significantly higher for children who subsequently developed epilepsy than in those who did not.

Hesdorffer et al. (2004) found that the risk of children to meet DSM-IV criteria for ADHD was 2.5 times higher than expected prior to the first spontaneous, unprovoked seizure. Jones et al. (2007) compared 53 children, aged 8 to 18 years, with recent-onset epilepsy, less than one-year duration, with a comparison group of 50 healthy children. The children with epilepsy had statistically significantly higher rates of depressive disorders (22.6% vs 4%), anxiety disorders (35.8% vs 22%) and attention deficit hyperactivity disorder (26.4% vs 10%). They also noted that a subset of children with epilepsy (45%) had DSM-IV Axis I disorders before the first recognised seizure. In addition to mood disorders, academic problems have been shown to be antecedents of childhood-onset epilepsy; about 25% of children were in need of special educational services even before the first diagnosed seizure (Oostrom et al., 2003; Hermann et al., 2006). Against this background, it is particularly interesting to note the findings of Saute et al., (2014) who reported decreased bilateral cortical thickness and decreased volume of subcortical and brainstem structures in children with new or recent-onset epilepsy and comorbid ADHD.

Rathouz et al. (2014) examined 69 children with new or recent-onset epilepsy shortly after diagnosis and five to six years later, with regard to intelligence, academic achievement, language, executive function and psychomotor speed, compared with 62 controls. Children with epilepsy performed significantly less well than their controls near the time of diagnosis; these findings persisted virtually unchanged over time, without progressive deterioration or recovery. The observations of Bonilha et al. (2014) on 39 children with new-onset epilepsy, compared with 28 healthy controls, suggested abnormal localized and bilateral hemispheric network organization with localization-related epilepsies and generalized epilepsies, respectively. In particular, children with epilepsy, low intelligence level and poor executive function had a suboptimal topographical structural organization with enhanced network segregation and reduced global integration. The same study group (Almane et al., 2014) showed that behavioural problems and lower social competence were significantly more common in children with new-onset epilepsy compared with controls, regardless of the type of syndrome.

Family clustering of behavioural disturbance in epilepsy

Hermann et al. (2012) paid attention to the aggregation of behavioural problems in families of children with epilepsy. There are several reports of disturbed cognitive performance and behaviour in family members (Oostrom et al., 2003; Hermann et al., 2006; Iqbal et al., 2009; Hesdorffer et al., 2012). This suggests that underlying genetic factors might be playing a role in causing both the behavioural disturbance and the epilepsy, although other factors, including environmental determinants, are certainly involved, at least in some cases. These important issues continue to be investigated.

Conclusions

Epidemiological studies in a number of different countries and over a long period of time have yielded reasonably consistent results with regard to the rates of psychiatric disorder in children with epilepsy, which have ranged from around 35% to 50%. The prevalence of psychiatric disorder in children with complicated epilepsy, usually implying accompanying intellectual disability, is much higher, well over 50%. Based on the findings of these studies, it is clear that psychiatric disorders in children with epilepsy represent a major issue and that good management of these disorders remains a major challenge.

References

Alfstad, K. A., Clench-Aas, J., Van, R. B., Mowinckel, P., Gjerstad, L. & Lossius, M. I. 2011. Psychiatric symptoms in Norwegian children with epilepsy aged 8-13 years: effects of age and gender? *Epilepsia*, 52, 1231-1238.

Almane, D., Jones, J. E., Jackson, D. C., Seidenberg, M. & Hermann, B. P. 2014. The social competence and behavioral problem substrate of new- and recent-onset childhood epilepsy. *Epilepsy Behav*, 31, 91-6.

Austin, J. K., Harezlak, J., Dunn, D. W., Huster, G. A., Rose, D. F. & Ambrosius, W. T. 2001. Behavior problems in children before first recognized seizures. *Pediatrics*, 107, 115-122.

Bjoernaes, H. 2001. Psychiatric comorbidity in epilepsy. *In*: JOHANNESSEN, S., TOMSON, T., SILLANPÄÄ, M. & PEDERSEN, B. (eds.) *Medical Risks in Epilepsy*. Petersfield, UK: Wrightson Biomedical Publishing.

Bonilha, L., Tabesh, A., Dabbs, K., Hsu, D. A., Stafstrom, C. E., Hermann, B. P. & Lin, J. J. 2014. Neurodevelopmental alterations of large-scale structural networks in children with new-onset epilepsy. *Hum Brain Mapp*, 35, 3661-72.

Bourgeois, B. F., Prensky, A. L., Palkes, H. S., Talent, B. K. & Busch, S. G. 1983. Intelligence in epilepsy: a prospective study in children. *Ann Neurol*, 14, 438-44.

Davies, S., Heyman, I. & Goodman, R. 2003. A population survey of mental health problems in children with epilepsy. *Developmental Medicine & Child Neurology*, 45, 292-295.

Dunn, D. W., Austin, J. K. & Huster, G. A. 1997. Behaviour problems in children with new-onset epilepsy. *Seizure*, 6, 283-287.

Fastenau, P. S., Johnson, C. S., Perkins, S. M., Byars, A. W., deGrauw, T. J., Austin, J. K. & Dunn, D. W. 2009. Neuropsychological status at seizure onset in children: risk factors for early cognitive deficits. *Neurology*, 73, 526-34.

Hermann, B., Jones, J., Sheth, R., Dow, C., Koehn, M. & Seidenberg, M. 2006. Children with new-onset epilepsy: neuropsychological status and brain structure. *Brain*, 129, 2609-19.

Hermann, B. P., Jones, J. E., Jackson, D. C. & Seidenberg, M. 2012. Starting at the beginning: the neuropsychological status of children with new-onset epilepsies. *Epileptic Disord*, 14, 12-21.

Hesdorffer, D. C., Caplan, R. & Berg, A. T. 2012. Familial clustering of epilepsy and behavioral disorders: evidence for a shared genetic basis. *Epilepsia*, 53, 301-307.

Hesdorffer, D. C., Ludvigsson, P., Olafsson, E., Gudmundsson, G., Kjartansson, O. & Hauser, W. A. 2004. ADHD as a risk factor for incident unprovoked seizures and epilepsy in children. *Archives of General Psychiatry*, 61, 731-736.

Hoare, P. 1984. The development of psychiatric disorder among schoolchildren with epilepsy. *Developmental Medicine & Child Neurology*, 26, 3-13.

Hoie, B., Sommerfelt, K., Waaler, P. E., Alsaker, F. D., Skeidsvoll, H. & Mykletun, A. 2008. The combined burden of cognitive, executive function, and psychosocial problems in children with epilepsy: a population-based study. *Developmental Medicine & Child Neurology*, 50, 530-536.

Hughes, J., Devinsky, O., Feldmann, E. & Bromfield, E. 1993. Premonitory symptoms in epilepsy. *Seizure*, 2, 201-3.

Iqbal, N., Caswell, H. L., Hare, D. J., Pilkington, O., Mercer, S. & Duncan, S. 2009. Neuropsychological profiles of patients with juvenile myoclonic epilepsy and their siblings: a preliminary controlled experimental video-EEG case series. *Epilepsy Behav.*, 14, 516-521.

Jalava, M., Sillanpää, M., Camfield, C. & Camfield, P. 1997. Social adjustment and competence 35 years after onset of childhood epilepsy: a prospective controlled study. *Epilepsia*, 38, 708-715.

Jones, J. E., Watson, R., Sheth, R., Caplan, R., Koehn, M., Seidenberg, M. & Hermann, B. 2007. Psychiatric comorbidity in children with new onset epilepsy. *Dev.Med.Child Neurol.*, 49, 493-497.

Long, C. G. & Moore, J. R. 1979. Parental expectations for their epileptic children. *J Child Psychol Psychiatry*, 20, 299-312.

McDermott, S., Mani, S. & Krishnaswami, S. 1995. A population-based analysis of specific behavior problems associated with childhood seizures. *Journal of Epilepsy*, 8, 110-118.

Oostrom, K. J., Smeets-Schouten, A., Kruitwagen, C. L., Peters, A. C., Jennekens-Schinkel, A. & Dutch Study Group of Epilepsy in, C. 2003. Not only a matter of epilepsy: early problems of cognition and behavior in children with "epilepsy only"--a prospective, longitudinal, controlled study starting at diagnosis. *Pediatrics*, 112, 1338-44.

Rantanen, K., Nieminen, P. & Eriksson, K. 2010. Neurocognitive functioning of preschool children with uncomplicated epilepsy. *J Neuropsychol*, 4, 71-87.

Rathouz, P. J., Zhao, Q., Jones, J. E., Jackson, D. C., Hsu, D. A., Stafstrom, C. E., Seidenberg, M. & Hermann, B. P. 2014. Cognitive development in children with new onset epilepsy. *Dev Med Child Neurol*, 56, 635-41.

Reilly, C., Atkinson, P., Das, K. B., Chin, R. F., Aylett, S. E., Burch, V., Gillberg, C., Scott, R. C. & Neville, B. G. 2014. Neurobehavioral comorbidities in children with active epilepsy: a population-based study. *Pediatrics*, 133, e1586-93.

Reilly, C., Atkinson, P., Das, K. B., Chin, R. F., Aylett, S. E., Burch, V., Gillberg, C., Scott, R. C. & Neville, B. G. 2015. Features of autism spectrum disorder (ASD) in childhood epilepsy: a population-based study. *Epilepsy & Behavior*, 42, 86-92.

Russ, S. A., Larson, K. & Halfon, N. 2012. A national profile of childhood epilepsy and seizure disorder. *Pediatrics*, 129, 256-264.

Rutter, M., Graham, P. & Yule, W. 1970. *A neuropsychiatric study in childhood*, London, Heinemann Medical.

Saute, R., Dabbs, K., Jones, J. E., Jackson, D. C., Seidenberg, M. & Hermann, B. P. 2014. Brain morphology in children with epilepsy and ADHD. *PLoS One*, 9, e95269.

Shackleton, D. P., Kasteleijn-Nolst Trenite, D. G., de Craen, A. J., Vandenbroucke, J. P. & Westendorp, R. G. 2003. Living with epilepsy: long-term prognosis and psychosocial outcomes. *Neurology*, 61, 64-70.

Sillanpää, M. 1987. Social adjustment and functioning of chronically ill and impaired children and adolescents. *Acta Paediatrica Scandinavica – Supplement*, 340, 1-70.

Sillanpää, M. 1992. Epilepsy in children: prevalence, disability, and handicap. *Epilepsia*, 33, 444-449.

Sillanpää, M. 2010. Long-term prognosis of adults with childhood rolandic epilepsy. *Journal of Epileptology*, 18.

Sillanpää, M., Jalava, M., Kaleva, O. & Shinnar, S. 1998. Long-term prognosis of seizures with onset in childhood. *New England Journal of Medicine*, 338, 1715-1722.

Speechley, K. N., Ferro, M. A., Camfield, C. S., Huang, W., Levin, S. D., Smith, M. L., Wiebe, S. & Zou, G. 2012. Quality of life in children with new-onset epilepsy: a 2-year prospective cohort study. *Neurology*, 79, 1548-1555.

Stores, G. 1978. School-children with epilepsy at risk for learning and behaviour problems. *Developmental Medicine & Child Neurology*, 20, 502-508.

World Health Organisation 1980. *International classification of impairments, disabilities, and handicaps: A manual of classification relating to the consequences of disease*, Geneva, ERIC Clearinghouse.

Epilepsy and ADHD

Frank Besag, Giuseppe Gobbi, Rochelle Caplan, Matti Sillanpää, Albert Aldenkamp, David W. Dunn

Abstract

ADHD occurs in about 30% of children with epilepsy. The causes of ADHD features include some antiepileptic drugs, the epilepsy itself and underlying brain dysfunction. Management of the ADHD will depend on the cause. Treatment with methylphenidate is effective in about 70% of cases; standard treatments with methylphenidate, dexamfetamine and atomoxetine are very unlikely to exacerbate seizures.

Key words: ADHD, epileptiform, Rolandic, antiepileptic

ADHD is one of the more common comorbidities of childhood epilepsy (Dunn, 2014; Salpekar and Mishra, 2014). It is typically reported in about 30% of children with epilepsy compared to 3-6% of controls (Davies *et al.*, 2003; Hermann *et al.*, 2007; Fastenau *et al.*, 2009; Russ *et al.*, 2012; Reilly *et al.*, 2014b). It also appears to be the most common disorder in both pre-school and school-age children with epilepsy (Socanski *et al.*, 2013), occurring equally in boys and girls, in contrast to the pattern in the general population, in which there is a predominance of boys. Approximately 70,000 school-age children in the UK have epilepsy and about 20,000 of these will have both epilepsy and ADHD. However, probably only a fraction are treated for the ADHD. Reluctance to treat may be related to diagnostic issues but is more likely to be related to concerns about possible seizure exacerbation.

■ Search strategy

In addition to studies already known to the authors, the Medline/PubMed database was searched from inception until the end of March 2015 using the search terms: epilep$ and (child$ or pediat$ or adolescen$) and (attention deficit or ADHD). Abstracts of likely relevance to the topic were examined to select papers for final detailed review. Reference lists of included papers were searched for any further relevant studies.

Epidemiology

Rate of ADHD in children with seizures

Hermann et al. (2007) studied 75 children aged 8-18 years with new or recent-onset idiopathic epilepsy and compared them with 62 controls. ADHD was found in 31% of the children with epilepsy and in 6% of the controls. Hesdorffer et al. (2004) carried out a population-based study in Icelandic children under 16 years of age. They found that ADHD was 2.5 times more common in children with newly-diagnosed, unprovoked seizures than in the controls. The ADHD was predominantly inattentive in type. Seizure type, frequency, aetiology or sex did not appear to be relevant factors. They suggested that there might be a common antecedent for both conditions. The study carried out by Dunn et al. (2003) was on a different population, namely those who had a history of epilepsy of at least six months duration. Of 175 children (90 male, 85 female), a total of 66 (38%) had ADHD of one type or another: 20 combined type, 42 predominantly inattentive type and four predominantly hyperactive-impulsive type. Again, there was an equal male to female ratio in the children with epilepsy and ADHD. Sherman et al. (2007) reported on a population of children with more severe epilepsy in a tertiary centre. Of 203 children, over 60% met screening criteria for ADHD. Of these, 40% had ADHD of the inattentive type and 18% of the hyperactive-impulsive type. Age of onset, epilepsy duration and seizure frequency did not appear to be related to the severity of inattention or hyperactivity-impulsivity.

More recently, Reilly et al. (2014a) found that, in a population of 85 children with active epilepsy, 80% had a DSM-IV-TR behavioral disorder and/or cognitive impairment. Intellectual disability (IQ < 70) (40%), ADHD (33%), and autism spectrum disorder (21%) were the most common neurobehavioral diagnoses.

Ku et al. (2014) reported that after 11 years of follow-up, the incidence rates of ADHD for a febrile seizure (FS) cohort and a control cohort were 7.83 and 4.72 per 1,000 person-years, respectively. The FS cohort was 1.66 times more at risk of ADHD occurrence (95% CI 1.27 to 2.18) than the control cohort. The risk of developing ADHD increased in conjunction with the frequency of FS-related visits. From a total of 198 children diagnosed with benign epilepsy with centrotemporal spikes (BECTS) at the Asan Medical Center, South Korea, Kim et al. (2014) reported that, in a cohort of 74 children (44 males) with neuropsychological examination, 48 (64.9%) had ADHD. A history of febrile convulsions was more common in patients with ADHD than in patients without ADHD ($p = 0.049$).

Zhang et al. (2014) investigated the prevalence of ADHD in 190 children with frontal lobe epilepsy, of whom 161 had effective follow up. Of these, 59% (95/161) had ADHD. They commented that 89.4% (76/85) of the children with abnormal EEG discharges on the most recent record had ADHD, whereas only 25% (19/76) with normal EEGs on the most recent record had ADHD.

Rate of epilepsy in children with ADHD

Davis et al. (2010), using the 1976-1982 Rochester birth cohort, identified 358 children with ADHD. Clinical data were available to age 20 for 81.3%. They found that children with ADHD were 2.7 times more likely to develop epilepsy than controls. Although this did not quite reach statistical significance ($p = 0.066$), the secondary analysis, when follow-up was censored at 18 years instead of 20 years, provided a higher proportion of clinical data (89% of cases) and in this analysis those with ADHD were 4.1 times more likely to have epilepsy than controls ($p = 0.022$, 95% confidence interval 1.23-13.52). Cohen et al. (2013) carried out a population-based study in Israel. The total study population was 284,419 children (mean age 9.4 years). The prevalence of epilepsy was 0.5% and the prevalence of ADHD 12.6%. Multivariate logistic regression with epilepsy as the dependent variable revealed an odds ratio for a child with ADHD having epilepsy of 2.4 (95% confidence interval 2.1-2.7).

Socanski et al. (2013) conducted a retrospective chart-review of children with ADHD who were evaluated between the years 2000 and 2005. Of 607 children with ADHD, 2.3% had a history of epilepsy; this is a higher rate than expected in the general paediatric population (0.5%). The majority of the patients had easily-treated epilepsy. All patients with epilepsy and ADHD were treated with methylphenidate (MPH); the initial response to MPH was 85.7%.

It should be noted that the overall results of these studies include children who had epilepsy before a diagnosis of ADHD as well as those in whom epilepsy was diagnosed after the diagnosis of ADHD. For example, in the study by Socanski et al. (2013), the diagnosis of epilepsy was made on average 1.8 years before the ADHD assessment.

Comorbid disorders

The rate of comorbidity in children who have either ADHD or epilepsy is high. Consequently, a high rate of comorbidity would also be expected in children who have both conditions. Gonzalez-Heydrich et al. (2007) found that 61% of 36 children with both epilepsy and ADHD, aged 6 to 17 years, had a comorbid disorder: 36% had anxiety disorders and 31% had oppositional defiant disorder. In this group of children, the combined subtype with both inattentive and hyperactive symptoms was the most frequent, occurring in 58%.

Possible causes of overactivity in children with epilepsy

There are many possible causes of the features of attention deficit hyperactivity disorder in children with epilepsy, including the following:
– "Classical" ADHD;
– Other psychiatric disorders;
– Associated/underlying brain damage or dysfunction;
– Causes related specifically to the epilepsy including:
  • Frequent epileptiform discharges: rolandic discharges, other focal discharges or generalised spike-wave discharges.
  • Postictal elevated mood.
  • Interictal manic psychosis.
– Adverse effects of medication.

"Classical" ADHD

As already stated, in epidemiological studies, a high proportion of children with epilepsy also have ADHD. The reason for this is debated but in most cases no other cause has been found and it has been concluded that the most likely explanation is an underlying factor causing both conditions (Hesdorffer et al., 2004). Some studies have reported that children with epilepsy are more likely to present with an inattentive form (Reilly, 2011) but this is not a universal finding.

Other psychiatric disorders

Other psychiatric disorders, not necessarily related to the epilepsy, may present with features of ADHD but careful assessment should distinguish them as being different. These disorders include conduct disorder, generalised anxiety disorder and elevated mood states such as hypomania or mania.

Associated/underlying brain damage or dysfunction

Associated underlying brain damage or dysfunction may include global developmental delay and specific frontal lobe damage or dysfunction. It is interesting to note that patients who may not present with the classical history of ADHD, including those with cerebral tumours, may nevertheless, in at least some cases, respond to the standard medication prescribed for this condition (Meyers et al., 1998).

Causes related specifically to the epilepsy

Frequent epileptiform discharges

Holtmann et al. (2003) examined the frequency of Rolandic spikes in the EEGs of 483 ADHD children, aged 2 to 16 years. Rolandic spikes were found in 27 (5.6%) of the ADHD children, which was significantly ($p = 0.001$) higher than the rate of 2.4% found in normal children (Cavazzuti et al., 1980). ADHD in the children with Rolandic spikes presented earlier; these children had more hyperactive-impulsive symptoms. In a further study, the same group (Holtmann et al., 2006) studied 48 children 6.7 to 14.9 years of age of whom 16 had ADHD and Rolandic spikes, 16 had ADHD without epileptiform discharges and 16 were healthy controls. The ADHD children with Rolandic spikes performed worse than the ADHD children without epileptiform discharges and healthy controls in a variety of tests. Rolandic spikes were associated with increased impulsivity, deficient inhibition and decreased interference control.

Socanski et al. (2010) examined EEGs from 517 out of a total of 607 children attending the only centre diagnosing and treating ADHD in an area of Norway. Epileptiform abnormalities were found in 39 (7.5%). Of these, 21 (53.9%) were generalised, 16 (41%) were focal and 2 (5.1%) had both focal and generalised abnormalities. Of the total group, nine (1.7%) had Rolandic spikes. A previous history of epileptic seizures was reported in 14 (2.5% of the children) and was more common in those who had epileptiform abnormalities.

It is interesting to note that Becker and Holtmann (2006) also reported that the EEGs of children with ADHD demonstrated increased theta activity and decreased alpha activity compared with normal controls. These changes are generally considered to be a non-specific indication of brain dysfunction.

Sinzig and Gontard (2005) analysed EEGs of 8,132 children and adolescents retrospectively. A new diagnosis of absence seizures was made in only 12 of these (0.44%) in the first centre and none in the second. They concluded that there was a minimal occurrence of absences in child and adolescent patients and that this was therefore not the main differential diagnosis that has to be considered in children with ADHD. However, they added that it was important to regard absence seizures as a rare differential diagnosis. Based on the experience of at least one of the current authors, in specialist centres, children certainly can present with ADHD symptoms because of very frequent absence seizures or epileptiform discharges.

Kanazawa (2014) found epileptiform discharges in 22.1% of 145 children with newly diagnosed ADHD for whom follow up was at least 3 months; those with IQ < 70 were excluded. Kim et al. (2014) reported that bilateral centrotemporal spikes on the EEG were more common in patients receiving ADHD medication than in patients with untreated ADHD ($p = 0.004$). Moreover, patients with frequent seizures prior to diagnosis and patients with a high spike index (≥ 40/min) on sleep EEG at diagnosis had significantly lower visual selective attention ($p < 0.05$). Children with BECTS had a high prevalence of ADHD; frequent seizures or interictal epileptiform abnormalities were closely related to impairment of visual selective attention. The authors concluded that there is the need for ADHD or attention-impairment screening in children with BECTS.

Elevated mood states

Children and teenagers who present with postictal elevated mood or interictal manic psychosis certainly have some features of ADHD. However, the history should distinguish clearly between these states and ADHD. For example, in the case of postictal elevated mood changes the history of recent seizures, typically a cluster, is characteristic and usually diagnostic. Above all, for both postictal and interictal elevated moods, the nature of the condition is intermittent, in contrast to the persistence of the ADHD symptoms. However, it should be noted that interictal elevated mood states may persist for long periods, for example several weeks or months (Kanemoto et al., 1996).

Antiepileptic drugs

Antiepileptic drugs, including the benzodiazepines (Sheth et al., 1994), phenobarbital (Domizio et al., 1993) and vigabatrin (Ferrie et al., 1996) can cause symptoms of ADHD in children, although there is a lack of consensus in the literature (see *Adverse cognitive and behavioural effects of antiepileptic drugs in children*, p. xx-xx). It is important to consider not only adverse effects of individual drugs but also adverse drug interactions. For example, if lamotrigine is added to carbamazepine in someone who is unable to express their experiences verbally and the patient develops diplopia and/or dizziness (Besag et al., 1998), they may present with distressed and overactive symptomatology. Treatment of these symptoms with ADHD medication would be entirely inappropriate; this situation can readily be resolved by decreasing the carbamazepine dose. Again, the history should distinguish this situation clearly from the ongoing symptoms of ADHD.

■ Should children with both epilepsy and ADHD be treated for the ADHD?

In the past there has been considerable reluctance to treat ADHD in the presence of epilepsy because of the concern of possible seizure exacerbations. Are these concerns justified by the evidence? What are the ADHD treatments of choice in children with both conditions?

The first step in the management of the child with epilepsy and ADHD must be to consider the possible causes already described. The management might need to be very different, depending on the cause. For example, if frequent absence seizures are causing the ADHD symptoms, additional or different antiepileptic medication may be appropriate. In contrast, if the child is overactive because of the adverse effects of antiepileptic medication, medication reductions or a change in antiepileptic medication rather than increasing antiepileptic medication will be appropriate.

If the diagnosis of ADHD is confirmed, the first-line treatment, regardless of whether the child has epilepsy or not, remains methylphenidate (MTA Cooperative Group, 1999). Controlled-release or extended-release methylphenidate has advantages in many children, based on the usual criteria: avoidance of peaks and troughs in effect and convenience of once-daily administration, although sometimes a top-up dose of methylphenidate is required later in the day. If methylphenidate is well-tolerated but not effective, there are theoretical reasons why dexamfetamine might be more effective (Faraone and Buitelaar, 2010). The second-line treatment is atomoxetine (Michelson et al., 2001). Third-line treatments include clonidine (Connor et al., 1999) and, particularly in children with learning disability and autism spectrum disorder in addition to the epilepsy, low-dose risperidone (Aman et al., 2004). Neither clonidine nor risperidone is licensed for treating ADHD in children but both may be of benefit. Clonidine is particularly valuable in children who have difficulty sleeping or who have a degree of oppositional-defiant disorder (Connor et al., 2000). This can be used in combination with methylphenidate; the reports of deaths with this combination were almost certainly not the result of the medication itself (Popper, 1995). Carbamazepine occasionally appears to be effective in the treatment of ADHD symptoms when other drugs have not been effective (Silva et al., 1996). It is not licensed for this indication.

How safe are these drugs for treating ADHD in children with epilepsy? What is the risk of seizure exacerbation? The British National Formulary (2013) states the following in relation to methylphenidate and dexamfetamine, respectively: "*caution – epilepsy (discontinue if increased seizure frequency) –*", "*caution – history of epilepsy (discontinue if convulsions occur) –*". What does the published evidence reveal with regard to possible seizure exacerbations?

One of the most frequently-quoted studies is that of Gross-Tsur et al. (1997) on 30 children with ADHD and epilepsy, aged 6.4 to 16.4 years. For the first two months they were treated with antiepileptic medication only. Methylphenidate was added in the next two months. None of the 25 children who were seizure-free had attacks with methylphenidate. Of five children with active seizures, three had an increase in seizures and the other two had no change or a reduction in seizures. There were no statistically significant changes in seizure control. If children with active epilepsy were treated with any additional medication, or indeed with no additional medication, the expected outcome would be that some might have fewer seizures, an approximately equal number would have more frequent seizures and some would have no change in seizure frequency. This is almost exactly the outcome that was reported in the study by Gross-Tsur et al. It would appear that no conclusions can be drawn from the study or, perhaps more accurately, it could be concluded that methylphenidate has no major effect on seizure control. The same authors also reported that there were no significant EEG changes with the methylphenidate and that, in terms of the ADHD symptoms, 70% derived benefit. They concluded that methylphenidate was effective in treating children with epilepsy and ADHD, and added that it was safe in children who were seizure-free. They commented that "*caution is warranted for those who are still having seizures while receiving AED therapy*", although it would appear that they had no evidence whatsoever from the results of their own study to support this statement.

Hemmer et al. (2001) presented results on 234 children with complicated ADHD of whom 36 (15.4%) had epileptiform abnormalities. 40% of the abnormal EEGs had Rolandic spikes. 60% of the abnormal EEGs had other focal abnormalities. 205 of the 234 (87.6%) were treated with stimulant medication. Seizures occurred only in the treated group; 1/175 patients with normal EEGs had seizures and 3/30, i.e. 10% (95% confidence interval 0%, 20.7%), with epileptiform discharges. Seizures occurred in two of the 12 children (16.7%) with Rolandic spikes. It is very difficult to draw any conclusions from these results other than that children with epileptiform abnormalities on the EEG are more likely to have seizures than those who do not, regardless of what treatment is given. The authors stated the following conclusions. *"These data suggest that a normal EEG can be used to assign children with ADHD to a category of minimal risk of seizure. In contrast an epileptiform EEG in neurologically normal children with ADHD predicts considerable risk for the eventual occurrence of seizure. The risk, however, is not necessarily attributable to stimulant use."* A similar conclusion might be drawn from the study by Socanski et al. (2013) (see earlier), who found that epileptiform abnormalities were more common in children with ADHD than in the general population, suggesting that children with ADHD are more at risk of having epilepsy.

Gucuyener et al. (2003) compared 57 patients who had ADHD and active seizures with 62 patients who had ADHD and EEG abnormalities before and after treatment with methylphenidate. They found that the seizure frequency did not change from baseline. The EEG appeared to improve, leading them to state that methylphenidate had a beneficial effect on the EEG. They concluded that methylphenidate is safe and effective in children with ADHD and concomitant active seizures or EEG abnormalities.

Santos et al. (2013) carried out a small study on 22 children (16 males, six females, mean age 11 years two months). An increased seizure frequency was noted in four patients, of whom one withdrew for this reason. After three months of treatment with methylphenidate, 73% no longer had clinically significant symptoms of ADHD. They reported that methylphenidate reduced the seizure severity. They concluded that low-dose methylphenidate was safe and effective in treating ADHD in resistant epilepsy, although it should be noted that results from a small study cannot necessarily be generalised to other populations.

There have been several reviews on ADHD and epilepsy (Dunn and Kronenberger, 2005; Baptista-Neto et al., 2008; Torres et al., 2008; Hamoda et al., 2009; Parisi et al., 2010), all of which have drawn broadly the same conclusions, namely that there is no evidence that methylphenidate causes seizure exacerbations when used to treat ADHD in people with epilepsy.

It can be concluded that both evidence and opinion suggests that previous concerns about methylphenidate causing seizure exacerbations in children with epilepsy and ADHD were probably not justified. Traditionally, dexamfetamine has been considered to be even less likely to worsen seizure control and it has even been suggested that it might improve seizure control.

Safety of other drug treatments for ADHD

Wernicke et al. (2007) reviewed two independent Eli Lilly databases: the Atomoxetine clinical trial base and the Atomoxetine post-marketing spontaneous adverse event database. The crude incidence rates of seizure adverse events were between 0.1 and 0.2%; there was no significant difference between atomoxetine and placebo. These authors concluded that, although children with ADHD are increasingly recognised as being at an elevated risk of seizures, treatment of the ADHD with atomoxetine does not appear to elevate this risk further. In a cohort study of the risk of seizures in a non-epilepsy paediatric population treated with atomoxetine, McAfee et al. (2013) compared 13,398 individuals initiated on atomoxetine with 13,322 initiated on stimulant medication and found no increased seizure risk with atomoxetine (relative risk 0.72, CI 0.37, 1.38). Torres et al. (2011), in a small study of 27 patients with epilepsy treated with atomoxetine, noted that there were no discontinuations because of seizure exacerbation. In another small study of 23 patients, Mulas et al. (2014) found no evidence of seizure exacerbation in children with epilepsy treated with stimulant or non-stimulant medication.

Risperidone is used in children with intellectual disability and behavioural problems who are often on the autism spectrum and have features of ADHD (Aman et al., 2004). Gonzalez-Heydrich et al. (2004) studied the seizure risk in 21 young people with epilepsy and psychiatric disorders, mean age 12 years, who were treated with risperidone 2.4 ± 3.5 mg/day. They reported that the psychiatric symptoms improved in 71% and the seizures were no worse in any patient.

Conclusions

– ADHD is under-diagnosed and under-treated in children with epilepsy.

– There is a broad differential diagnosis for the causes of ADHD symptoms in children with epilepsy, including the epilepsy itself and some antiepileptic drugs. The management of ADHD in the child with epilepsy will depend on the cause.

– Approximately 30% of children with epilepsy have ADHD and about 70% of children with ADHD and epilepsy will benefit from standard treatment such as methylphenidate; there appears to be no firm evidence that the usual treatments for ADHD are likely to exacerbate seizures.

References

Aman, M. G., Binder, C. & Turgay, A. 2004. Risperidone effects in the presence/absence of psychostimulant medicine in children with ADHD, other disruptive behavior disorders, and subaverage IQ. *Journal of child and adolescent psychopharmacology*, 14, 243-254.

Baptista-Neto, L., Dodds, A., Rao, S., Whitney, J., Torres, A. & Gonzalez-Heydrich, J. 2008. An expert opinion on methylphenidate treatment for attention deficit hyperactivity disorder in pediatric patients with epilepsy. *Expert Opinion on Investigational Drugs*, 17, 77-84.

Becker, K. & Holtmann, M. 2006. Role of electroencephalography in attention-deficit hyperactivity disorder. *Expert Review of Neurotherapeutics*, 6, 731-739.

Besag, F. M. C., Berry, D. J., Pool, F., Newbery, J. E. & Subel, B. 1998. Carbamazepine toxicity with lamotrigine: pharmacokinetic or pharmacodynamic interaction? *Epilepsia*, 39, 183-187.

Cavazzuti, G. B., Cappella, L. & Nalin, A. 1980. Longitudinal study of epileptiform EEG patterns in normal children. *Epilepsia*, 21, 43-55.

Cohen, R., Senecky, Y., Shuper, A., Inbar, D., Chodick, G., Shalev, V. & Raz, R. 2013. Prevalence of Epilepsy and Attention-Deficit Hyperactivity (ADHD) Disorder A Population-Based Study. *Journal of Child Neurology*, 28, 120-123.

Connor, D. F., Barkley, R. A. & Davis, H. T. 2000. A pilot study of methyiphenidate, clonidine, or the combination in ADHD comorbid with aggressive oppositional defiant or conduct disorder. *Clinical Pediatrics*, 39, 15-25.

Connor, D. F., Fletcher, K. E. & Swanson, J. M. 1999. A meta-analysis of clonidine for symptoms of attention-deficit hyperactivity disorder. *Journal of the American Academy of Child & Adolescent Psychiatry*, 38, 1551-1559.

Davies, S., Heyman, I. & Goodman, R. 2003. A population survey of mental health problems in children with epilepsy. *Developmental Medicine & Child Neurology*, 45, 292-295.

Davis, S. M., Katusic, S. K., Barbaresi, W. J., Killian, J., Weaver, A. L., Ottman, R. & Wirrell, E. C. 2010. Epilepsy in Children with ADHD: A Population-Based Study. *Pediatric Neurology*, 42, 325.

Domizio, S., Verrotti, A., Ramenghi, L. A., Sabatino, G. & Morgese, G. 1993. Anti-epileptic therapy and behaviour disturbances in children. *Childs Nerv.Syst.*, 9, 272-274.

Dunn, D. W. 2014. Focusing on ADHD and attention in children with epilepsy. *Epilepsy Behav*, 37, 308-9.

Dunn, D. W., Austin, J. K., Harezlak, J. & Ambrosius, W. T. 2003. ADHD and epilepsy in childhood. *Developmental Medicine & Child Neurology*, 45, 50-54.

Dunn, D. W. & Kronenberger, W. G. 2005. Childhood epilepsy, attention problems, and ADHD: review and practical considerations. *Seminars in Pediatric Neurology*, 12, 222-228.

Faraone, S. V. & Buitelaar, J. 2010. Comparing the efficacy of stimulants for ADHD in children and adolescents using meta-analysis. *European child & adolescent psychiatry*, 19, 353-364.

Fastenau PS, Johnson CS, Perkins SM, et al. 2009. Neuropsychological status at seizure onset in children: risk factors for early cognitive deficits. *Neurology*, 73, 526-34.

Ferrie, C. D., Robinson, R. O. & Panayiotopoulos, C. P. 1996. Psychotic and severe behavioural reactions with vigabatrin: a review. *Acta Neurologica Scandinavica*, 93, 1-8.

Gonzalez-Heydrich, J., Dodds, A., Whitney, J., MacMillan, C., Waber, D., Faraone, S. V., Boyer, K., Mrakotsky, C., DeMaso, D., Bourgeois, B. & Biederman, J. 2007. Psychiatric disorders and behavioral characteristics of pediatric patients with both epilepsy and attention-deficit hyperactivity disorder. *Epilepsy & Behavior*, 10, 384-388.

Gonzalez-Heydrich, J., Pandina, G. J., Fleisher, C. A., Hsin, O., Raches, D., Bourgeois, B. F. & Biederman, J. 2004. No seizure exacerbation from risperidone in youth with comorbid epilepsy and psychiatric disorders: a case series. *Journal of Child & Adolescent Psychopharmacology*, 14, 295-310.

Gross-Tsur, V., Manor, O., van der, M. J., Joseph, A. & Shalev, R. S. 1997. Epilepsy and attention deficit hyperactivity disorder: is methylphenidate safe and effective? *Journal of Pediatrics*, 130, 670-674.

Gucuyener, K., Erdemoglu, A. K., Senol, S., Serdaroglu, A., Soysal, S. & Kockar, A. I. 2003. Use of methylphenidate for attention-deficit hyperactivity disorder in patients with epilepsy or electroencephalographic abnormalities. *Journal of Child Neurology*, 18, 109-112.

Hamoda, H. M., Guild, D. J., Gumlak, S., Travers, B. H. & Gonzalez-Heydrich, J. 2009. Association between attention-deficit/hyperactivity disorder and epilepsy in pediatric populations. *Expert Review of Neurotherapeutics*, 9, 1747-1754.

Hemmer, S. A., Pasternak, J. F., Zecker, S. G. & Trommer, B. L. 2001. Stimulant therapy and seizure risk in children with ADHD. *Pediatric Neurology*, 24, 99-102.

Hermann, B., Jones, J., Dabbs, K., Allen, C. A., Sheth, R., Fine, J., McMillan, A. & Seidenberg, M. 2007. The frequency, complications and aetiology of ADHD in new onset paediatric epilepsy. *Brain*, 130, 12-48.

Hesdorffer, D. C., Ludvigsson, P., Olafsson, E., Gudmundsson, G., Kjartansson, O. & Hauser, W. A. 2004. ADHD as a risk factor for incident unprovoked seizures and epilepsy in children. *Archives of General Psychiatry*, 61, 731-736.

Holtmann, M., Becker, K., Kentner-Figura, B. & Schmidt, M. H. 2003. Increased frequency of rolandic spikes in ADHD children. *Epilepsia*, 44, 1241-1244.

Holtmann, M., Matei, A., Hellmann, U., Becker, K., Poustka, F. & Schmidt, M. H. 2006. Rolandic spikes increase impulsivity in ADHD – a neuropsychological pilot study. *Brain & Development*, 28, 633-640.

Kanazawa, O. 2014. Reappraisal of abnormal EEG findings in children with ADHD: on the relationship between ADHD and epileptiform discharges. *Epilepsy Behav*, 41, 251-6.

Kanemoto, K., Kawasaki, J. & Kawai, I. 1996. Postictal psychosis: a comparison with acute interictal and chronic psychoses. *Epilepsia*, 37, 551-6.

Kim, E. H., Yum, M. S., Kim, H. W. & Ko, T. S. 2014. Attention-deficit/hyperactivity disorder and attention impairment in children with benign childhood epilepsy with centrotemporal spikes. *Epilepsy Behav*, 37, 54-8.

Ku, Y. C., Muo, C. H., Ku, C. S., Chen, C. H., Lee, W. Y., Shen, E. Y., Chang, Y. J. & Kao, C. H. 2014. Risk of subsequent attention deficit-hyperactivity disorder in children with febrile seizures. *Arch Dis Child*, 99, 322-6.

McAfee, A. T., Landon, J., Jones, M., Bangs, M. E., Acharya, N., Hornbuckle, K. & Wong, J. 2013. A cohort study of the risk of seizures in a pediatric population treated with atomoxetine or stimulant medications. *Pharmacoepidemiol Drug Saf*, 22, 386-93.

Meyers, C. A., Weitzner, M. A., Valentine, A. D. & Levin, V. A. 1998. Methylphenidate therapy improves cognition, mood, and function of brain tumor patients. *Journal of Clinical Oncology*, 16, 2522-2527.

Michelson D, Faries D, Wernicke J, et al. 2001. Atomoxetine in the treatment of children and adolescents with attention-deficit/hyperactivity disorder: a randomized, placebo-controlled, dose-response study. *Pediatrics*, 108, E83.

MTA Cooperative Group 1999. A 14-month randomized clinical trial of treatment strategies for attention-deficit/hyperactivity disorder. *Archives of General Psychiatry*, 56, 1073.

Mulas, F., Roca, P., Ros-Cervera, G., Gandia-Beneto, R. & Ortiz-Sanchez, P. 2014. Pharmacological management of attention deficit hyperactivity disorder with methylphenidate and atomoxetine within a context of epilepsy. *Rev Neurol*, 58 Suppl 1, S43-9.

Parisi, P., Moavero, R., Verrotti, A. & Curatolo, P. 2010. Attention deficit hyperactivity disorder in children with epilepsy. *Brain & Development*, 32, 10-16.

Popper, C. W. 1995. Combining methylphenidate and clonidine: pharmacologic questions and news reports about sudden death. *Journal of Child and Adolescent Psychopharmacology*, 5, 157-166.

Reilly, C., Atkinson, P., Das, K. B., Chin, R. F., Aylett, S. E., Burch, V., Gillberg, C., Scott, R. C. & Neville, B. G. 2014a. Neurobehavioral comorbidities in children with active epilepsy: a population-based study. *Pediatrics*, 133, e1586-93.

Reilly C, Atkinson P, Das KB, et al. 2014b. Screening for mental health disorders in active childhood epilepsy: population-based data. *Epilepsy Research*, 108, 1917-26.

Reilly, C. J. 2011. Attention deficit hyperactivity disorder (ADHD) in childhood epilepsy. *Research in Developmental Disabilities*, 32, 883-893.

Royal Pharmaceutical Society of Great Britain 2013. *British National Formulary*, London, BMJ Group and Pharmaceutical Press, Royal Pharmaceutical Society.

Russ, S. A., Larson, K. & Halfon, N. 2012. A national profile of childhood epilepsy and seizure disorder. *Pediatrics*, 129, 256-264.

Salpekar, J. A. & Mishra, G. 2014. Key issues in addressing the comorbidity of attention deficit hyperactivity disorder and pediatric epilepsy. *Epilepsy Behav*, 37, 310-5.

Santos K, Palmini A, Radziuk AL, et al. 2013. The impact of methylphenidate on seizure frequency and severity in children with attention-deficit-hyperactivity disorder and difficult-to-treat epilepsies. *Developmental Medicine & Child Neurology*, 55, 654-660.

Sherman, E. M., Slick, D. J., Connolly, M. B. & Eyrl, K. L. 2007. ADHD, neurological correlates and health-related quality of life in severe pediatric epilepsy. *Epilepsia*, 48, 1083-1091.

Sheth, R. D., Goulden, K. J. & Ronen, G. M. 1994. Aggression in children treated with clobazam for epilepsy. *Clinical Neuropharmacology*, 17, 332-337.

Silva, R. R., Munoz, D. M. & Alpert, M. 1996. Carbamazepine use in children and adolescents with features of attention-deficit hyperactivity disorder: a meta-analysis. *J Am Acad Child Adolesc Psychiatry*, 35, 352-8.

Sinzig, J. K. & von Gontard, A. 2005. Absences as differential diagnosis in children with attention-deficit disorder [German]. *Klinische Pädiatrie*, 217, 230-233.

Socanski, D., Aurlien, D., Herigstad, A., Thomsen, P. H. & Larsen, T. K. 2013. Epilepsy in a large cohort of children diagnosed with attention deficit/hyperactivity disorders (ADHD). *Seizure.*, 22, 651-655.

Socanski, D., Herigstad, A., Thomsen, P. H., Dag, A. & Larsen, T. K. 2010. Epileptiform abnormalities in children diagnosed with attention deficit/hyperactivity disorder. *Epilepsy Behav.*, 19, 483-486.

Torres, A., Whitney, J., Rao, S., Tilley, C., Lobel, R. & Gonzalez-Heydrich, J. 2011. Tolerability of atomoxetine for treatment of pediatric attention-deficit/hyperactivity disorder in the context of epilepsy. *Epilepsy Behav*, 20, 95-102.

Torres, A. R., Whitney, J. & Gonzalez-Heydrich, J. 2008. Attention-deficit/hyperactivity disorder in pediatric patients with epilepsy: review of pharmacological treatment. *Epilepsy & Behavior*, 12, 217-233.

Wernicke, J. F., Holdridge, K. C., Jin, L., Edison, T., Zhang, S., Bangs, M. E., Allen, A. J., Ball, S. & Dunn, D. 2007. Seizure risk in patients with attention-deficit-hyperactivity disorder treated with atomoxetine. *Developmental Medicine & Child Neurology*, 49, 498-502.

Zhang, D. Q., Li, F. H., Zhu, X. B. & Sun, R. P. 2014. Clinical observations on attention-deficit hyperactivity disorder (ADHD) in children with frontal lobe epilepsy. *J Child Neurol*, 29, 54-7.

Epilepsy and autism

Frank Besag, Albert Aldenkamp, Rochelle Caplan,
David W. Dunn, Giuseppe Gobbi, Matti Sillanpää

Abstract

A high proportion of children with epilepsy have autism spectrum disorder. Although estimates vary, depending both on the population studied and the definitions used, a figure of around 20% has typically been reported. Autism can have a major impact on the life of the child and family. Despite the importance of this comorbidity and although many studies have been performed, a full understanding of the possible links between epilepsy and autism remains elusive. In a minority of cases, for example in the Landau-Kleffner syndrome, the autistic features can be the result of the epilepsy itself. However, there has been a failure to demonstrate that the epilepsy itself plays a major role in most cases. The current evidence seems to point to a common underlying predisposing factor. The discovery of a growing number of genetic defects leading to both conditions would support this explanation of the link.

Key words: autism, ESES, CSWS, epileptiform

■ Search strategy

In addition to studies already known to the authors, the Medline/PubMed database was searched from inception until the end of March 2015 using the search terms: epilep$ and (child$ or pediat$ or adolescen$) and (autism or autistic). Abstracts of likely relevance to the topic were examined to select papers for final detailed review. Reference lists of included papers were searched for any further relevant studies.

■ Epidemiology

The prevalence of epilepsy in childhood is around 4-7 per 1,000 (Sillanpää, 1992) and the prevalence of autism spectrum disorder (ASD) is approximately 1% (Baird *et al.*, 2006b). Estimates of the prevalence of epilepsy in autism range widely, from approximately 2 to 40% (Woolfenden *et al.*, 2012), depending not only on the group of subjects studied but also on the criteria and ascertainment used both for the diagnosis of epilepsy and, particularly, the diagnosis of autism/ASD. Furthermore, the prevalence will depend on the age at which the subjects are studied. There are two peaks of onset of epilepsy associated with autism, the first in infancy and the second in the teenage years. This implies that the childhood prevalence is likely to be lower than the prevalence in the late teenage years. Some studies quote point prevalence and others quote lifetime prevalence; the latter will clearly be higher. The rate of misdiagnosis of epilepsy is high, typically around 20-25% (Jeavons, 1983; Uldall et al., 2006). The diagnosis of autism is subjective, since there is no laboratory test for the condition. Interviews, questionnaires and observational instruments are all subject to error. Most of the studies on the prevalence of autism and epilepsy have not been prospective and have been on selected samples, rather than being population studies. The prevalence of autism also depends very much on the level of intellectual ability (Amiet et al., 2008).

Steffenburg et al. (1995) carried out a population study in Goteborg, Sweden, on cohorts of children aged 6-9 years and 10-13 years. Ninety-eight children met the criteria for intellectual disability (mental retardation) and active epilepsy. Twenty-four subjects (27%) had "autistic disorder" and a further 10 (11%) had "an autistic-like condition". Of the 90 children examined, 53 (57%) had at least one additional psychiatric diagnosis, the most common being ADHD. A subsequent study by the same group (Steffenburg et al., 1996) showed that the prevalence of autism increased with age, up to 10 years. At 10 years, the prevalence of autism alone was 8%, of autism with severe mental retardation but no cerebral palsy 27% and autism with severe mental retardation and cerebral palsy 67%. Clarke et al. (2005) based a diagnosis of autism on the autism screening questionnaire (ASQ) in a tertiary care clinic. Of the 97 ASQ questionnaires that were properly completed, 32% fulfilled the criteria for ASD. The children in this study were aged 2-18 years (mean age 12.7 years). However, the questionnaire return rate was only one-third, implying that the results might not have been typical of the whole sample of children attending the clinic. Danielsson et al. (2005) carried out a further study on the population of individuals identified with epilepsy born from 1962 to 1984 in Goteborg. They found that 30% of 120 individuals with autistic disorder or "autistic-like condition" had epilepsy at some point in their lives. By the time of this study, six (5%) of the 120 individuals had died and six (5%) had parents who did not want to participate. The remaining 108 subjects (77 male and 31 female, mean age at study 25.5 years, range 17-40 years) were included. Amiet et al. (2008) reviewed all data available from published reports from 1963 to 2006 on autism and epilepsy. They carried out meta-analyses and found that the pooled prevalence of epilepsy was 21.5% in autistic subjects with intellectual disability compared to 8% in those without intellectual disability. The male to female ratio of autism with epilepsy was approximately 2:1 in contrast to the male to female ratio of autism without epilepsy which was 3.5:1. Epilepsy was more likely to occur in girls with autism ($p < 0.001$). Turk et al. (2009) compared two groups of 60 children, aged 7-17 years, with autism spectrum disorder: one with epilepsy (ASD + epilepsy) and the other without (ASD only). The male to female ratio was 6.5:1 in the ASD-only group but only 2:1 in the ASD + epilepsy group. The group with ASD + epilepsy were more likely to have had a later diagnosis of ASD and, in contrast to what might have been expected, were no more likely to be aloof and passive than the ASD-only group. As might have been predicted, the ASD + epilepsy group had more motor difficulties, developmental delays and challenging behaviours, in keeping with previous findings. Although the investigators endeavoured to recruit all children with autism in a given geographical area, the groups were not very well matched, implying that the results cannot confidently be generalised to other populations.

Berg et al. (2011) carried out a community-based, prospective, long-term, follow-up study of children enrolled when first diagnosed with epilepsy by paediatric neurologists in the state of Connecticut from 1993 to 1997. Parents were interviewed at five and nine years after the initial recruitment into the study. For the majority of the children (489/613), an interview was carried out at both these times. In addition, medical and other records were scrutinised. It should be noted, however, that no standard autism screening instrument was used, nor were the children examined personally to determine whether they had autism. Twenty-eight were classified as definitely or probably having ASD, 26 by parental interview and two through medical records only. One of the children had Rett syndrome and all of the 28 had ASD before the onset of epilepsy. In another 24 children the diagnosis (although not necessarily the initial onset of symptoms) of ASD was identified after the children had been recognised as having epilepsy. There were a further 28 children who were identified by the parent or from the medical records as having possible ASD that were excluded on further scrutiny. A further 21 children had autism-spectrum-disorder-like features but did not have definite or possible ASD. The overall prevalence of ASD was 5% (95% confidence interval 3.2-6.9%). In those with an estimated IQ of 80 or greater, the prevalence was 2.2% (95% confidence interval 0.8-3.6%) compared with 13.8% (95% confidence interval 8-19.5%) in those who had an IQ of less than 80. In the bivariate analysis, male gender, early age of onset, IQ less than 80 and West syndrome were all associated with ASD. The same parameters, apart from West syndrome, were all associated with autistic-like features. On the basis of multiple logistic regression, the following characteristics were correlated with ASD in 27 of these children with this diagnosis (excluding the one child with Rett syndrome): a history of West syndrome, prevalence ratio 3.4, 95% confidence interval 1.36-8.65, $p = 0.009$, intellectual impairment, prevalence ratio 5.08, 95% confidence interval 2.15-12.0, $p = 0.0002$ and male sex, prevalence ratio 2.22, 95% confidence interval 0.97-5.07, $p = 0.06$. The following factors were independently associated with ASD in children with no history of West syndrome: intellectual impairment, prevalence ratio 4.46, 95% confidence interval 1.93-11.25, $p = 0.0006$ and male sex, prevalence ratio 3.71, 95% confidence interval 1.24-11.1, $p = 0.02$. The authors concluded that West syndrome appeared to have a strong and specific association with ASD. Apart from this association, the main risk factors for ASD in children with epilepsy seemed to be the same as in the general population, although there did appear to be a small increased risk of this disorder associated with childhood-onset epilepsy in the absence of cognitive impairment. However, it should be noted that the numbers, when stratified, were quite small and the confidence interval for ASD occurring in those with an IQ of more than 80 was 0.8-3.6%; this implies that, although the prevalence was 2.2%, which is higher than the most recent estimates of autism prevalence in whole population studies, the confidence interval overlaps with the figure for autism in the general population.

Matsuo et al. (2010) studied 519 patients with epilepsy, aged 2-43 years (median 11 years), followed up at the paediatric department of a children's hospital. All of these patients had the first seizure before 18 years of age. Seventy-nine patients (15.2%) had ASD, which included autism, Asperger syndrome and pervasive developmental disorder not otherwise specified (PDD-NOS). The most frequent age of onset of seizures was 4 years. The epilepsy onset was before 10 years of age in 85%. ASD was detected after the onset of epilepsy in 47%. The authors pointed out that eight of these 29 cases had been overlooked for more than five years; most of these had high-functioning ASD. The most frequent seizure type was complex partial (dyscognitive) seizures (68%). Paroxysmal

EEG abnormalities in the frontal area were recorded in about half of the cases. They concluded that complex partial (dyscognitive) seizures with frontal paroxysms occurring from 1 to 9 years of age seemed to be characteristic of epilepsy associated with ASD. They also drew attention to the fact that their study did not show a second peak of epilepsy onset in teenagers with ASD but this was because the clinics were mainly for children of less than 15 years of age. The male to female ratio of idiopathic ASD was 3 to 1 and of secondary ASD was 2.4 to 1. They stated that this was consistent with other studies suggesting that epilepsy might be more prevalent in females with ASD than in males with ASD because these ratios are lower than the male to female ratio of autism quoted for the general population.

Bolton (2011) carried out a long-term follow-up study of individuals who were diagnosed with autism in childhood. The study was performed when the subjects were at least 21 years of age. Of this group of 150 individuals, 22% had developed epilepsy, the majority after 10 years of age. However, it should be noted that those with a history of infantile spasms or those with severe or profound intellectual disability (mental retardation) were excluded. The group with epilepsy was compared to those in the same clinic population who did not develop epilepsy. Both verbal and non-verbal ability were lower in the epilepsy group. As in other studies, the gender ratio was more equal in those with epilepsy (39% female) than in those without epilepsy (24% female).

Jokiranta et al. (2014) identified cases of autism spectrum disorder through the Finnish Prenatal Study of Autism and Autism Spectrum Disorders, which included data on 4,705 children. They examined associations between epilepsy and various types of autism spectrum disorder, including childhood autism, Asperger syndrome and pervasive developmental disorders (not otherwise specified). Each case was matched to four controls. They found that epilepsy was associated with autism spectrum disorder in all of the autism spectrum disorder groups, after adjusting for covariates. However, the association was stronger in the group with intellectual disability, especially females.

Woolfenden et al. (2012) carried out a systematic review of two outcomes in autism spectrum disorder: epilepsy and mortality. They found 16 studies in which the percentage of those with autism who had developed epilepsy was measured after at least 12 months of observation. In two of the studies, for which the age at follow-up was under 12 years, the majority of subjects did not have intellectual disability and the estimate of the percentage having epilepsy at follow-up was 6.1% (95% confidence interval 3.8-9.0%). In nine of the studies, the majority of subjects did have intellectual disability and the age at follow-up was 12 years or more; the pooled estimate of the percentage having epilepsy at follow-up was 23.7% (95% confidence interval 17.5-30.5%). It is interesting to note that these figures are very comparable with the previous analysis by Amiet et al. (2008), namely 8% and 21.5%, respectively (see earlier). Woolfenden et al. also examined the effect of gender; three papers provided this data: 3-10% of females had epilepsy compared to 13-29% of males.

Causes of autism in children with epilepsy

This subject has been discussed by a number of authors, notably Tuchman and co-workers (Tuchman et al., 2010; Tuchman and Cuccaro, 2011; Cuccaro et al., 2012; Tuchman, 2013). As previously discussed (Besag, 2009), the cause of the link between epilepsy and autism might be framed in the following three questions.

- Can epilepsy result in autistic features?
- Can autism cause epilepsy?
- Could there be underlying causes or conditions that predispose both to autism and epilepsy?

These questions will be discussed in turn.

Can epilepsy result in autistic features?

There are many anecdotal reports of this, demonstrated clearly by the resolution or reduction of autistic features when the epilepsy, manifesting as seizures and/or epileptiform abnormalities, is treated successfully – see later. One of the reasons that there has been such an intense interest in the possibility that epilepsy might play a role in the causation of autism is the finding that 15-40% of children with autism regress, *i.e.* lose skills, within the first three years of life, raising the question of whether some subtle manifestation of epilepsy might be playing a role (Baird *et al.*, 2008). Although the rate of epileptiform abnormality in the EEG of subjects with autism is high, there seems to be no association with regression, as demonstrated by Chez *et al.* (2006). They carried out a retrospective review of 24-hour ambulatory EEG data from 889 patients with autism spectrum disorder and found that 540 (60.7%) had abnormal epileptiform activity in sleep. The epileptiform discharges were most frequently localised over the right temporal region. Eighty of 176 patients treated with valproic acid had normalisation of the EEG and an additional 30 showed improvement on the EEG. As discussed in the paper on epilepsy syndromes (see later), Roulet-Perez *et al.* (1993) described an acquired epileptic frontal syndrome in four children with continuous spike waves in slow-wave sleep (CSWS) who had mental and behavioural regression. They commented that the pattern of behavioural and cognitive disturbance was similar to that found in some autistic-like disorders but they also drew attention to the similarity to the features of frontal lobe syndrome, more commonly described in adults. Deonna and Roulet (2006) have stated that it is disappointing that after a period of 10-20 years during which there has been a hope of finding epilepsy as a possible cause of autism there has been a growing absence of evidence of a direct causal link. Tharp (2004) reviewed the data and concluded that there was no justification to support the use of antiepileptic medication or surgery in children with pervasive developmental disorders, *i.e.* that there is no evidence that treatment to eliminate EEG spikes would have a therapeutic effect on the behavioural abnormalities of autism. Baird *et al.* (2006a) carried out an audit of sleep EEGs in 64 children (18-48 months) with autism, none of whom had a history suggestive of epilepsy. Thirty-nine had regressive autism. Twenty showed some epileptiform abnormality. Although the authors found that there was no statistically significant difference in epileptiform activity in those who showed regression compared with those who did not, it should be noted that the percentage of abnormal EEGs was higher (38.5%) in those who had set-back compared with those who did not (20%) and, although the overall difference was not statistically significant ($p = 0.07$), the p value was not far above 0.05, raising the possibility that larger numbers might have revealed a statistically significant difference.

There are major methodological difficulties in endeavouring to assess the role of epileptiform discharges in autistic regression. A daytime EEG may not pick up abnormalities that are clinically significant. Twenty-four-hour monitoring or, at least, sleep monitoring is recommended. Furthermore, if the regression takes place over a short period of time and the EEG is carried out after the period of regression, it would not be surprising if the EEG abnormality were largely "burnt out" by that stage, resulting in a false negative result. This area, which has been one of great controversy, remains open to debate.

Can autism cause epilepsy?

The second possibility is that autism might cause epilepsy. No reasonable hypothesis appears to have been put forward to suggest causality in this direction.

Could there be underlying causes or conditions that predispose both to autism and epilepsy?

The third possibility is that there is an underlying disorder or abnormality leading both to epilepsy and to autism (Brooks-Kayal, 2010; Tuchman and Cuccaro, 2011). The finding that the majority of children with epilepsy who have autism are also in the intellectual disability range (IQ less than 70) offers strong supportive evidence to this suggestion. However, it should be noted that, as indicated earlier, there appears to be a small increase in epilepsy in those who have autism but do not have intellectual disability (Amiet et al., 2008). More recent genetic work suggests that a number of gene defects might be associated both with epilepsy and autism. This issue has been discussed in some detail by Tuchman and Cuccaro (2011). Particular attention should be drawn to the review by Betancur (2011), which has the thought-provoking title *Etiological heterogeneity in autism spectrum disorders: more than 100 genetic and genomic disorders and still counting*. In that review, data is provided on 103 disease genes and 44 genomic loci reported in subjects with autism spectrum disorder or autistic behaviour. She points out that these genes and loci have all been causally implicated in intellectual disability, indicating that these two conditions share a common genetic basis. Furthermore, she has made the important point that the findings illustrate that autism is not a single condition. She reports that the most common single gene mutation in subjects with autism spectrum disorders is Fragile X syndrome (FMR1), present in about 2% of cases. A number of other monogenetic disorders in which ASD can occur include tuberous sclerosis (TSC1, TSC2), neurofibromatosis (NF1), Angelman syndrome (UBE3A), Rett syndrome (MECP2) and PTEN mutations associated with macrocephaly and autism. Rare mutations identified in synaptic genes include NLGN3, NLGN4X, SHANK3 and SHANK. A large number of other genetic disorders are included in that review. Particular attention has been drawn to copy number variants (CNVs). These can include microdeletions and microduplications with variable expressivity and/or incomplete penetrance. Those associated with neurodevelopmental disorders include 1q21.1, 15q13.3, 16p13.11, 16p11.2 and 22q11.2.

What conclusions can be drawn about the cause of autism? The first conclusion should be that the search for a single cause is unlikely to be successful, regardless of whether the subjects have epilepsy or not, since autism, as already stated, appears to represent a number of different conditions with common clinical characteristics. There are likely to be multiple causes but identifying at least some of these might be helpful in management.

■ The management of children with epilepsy and autism

The management of the child with epilepsy and autism basically consists of managing each of these conditions as they would be managed on their own, with certain notable exceptions. Rarely, a child may lose skills because of electrical status epilepticus of slow wave sleep (ESES)/continuous spike-waves in slow-wave sleep (CSWS). As stated in previous reviews, although the Landau-Kleffner syndrome of acquired epileptic aphasia is a rare condition, it provides an interesting model in this context, since it is reported that 20-30% of these children do not have obvious seizures (Caraballo et al., 2014). Despite this, antiepileptic treatment with medication or with surgery such as multiple subpial transection (Morrell et al., 1989) can be highly effective if implemented early. ESES/CSWS does not always present with regression of language skills; it may present with loss of other skills. Again, treatment to abolish the epileptiform abnormality may result in partial or substantial return of the lost skills. Apart from these important exceptions, standard management for both epilepsy and autism spectrum disorder should be implemented. Notwithstanding these comments, Robinson (2012) has pointed out that there are several reports of reductions in emotional lability, aggression, impulsivity and self-injurious behaviour with a number of antiepileptic drugs including carbamazepine (Gillberg, 1991), valproic acid (Nass and Petrucha, 1990; Plioplys, 1994; Childs and Blair, 1997), divalproex sodium (Hollander et al., 2006), lamotrigine (Uvebrant and Bauziene, 1994) and topiramate (Hardan et al., 2004). However, most of these reports are single cases or open trials. Although the study by Hollander et al. (2006) was a double-blind, placebo-controlled trial of divalproex sodium against placebo, the number of participants with autism spectrum disorder (13) was small and the duration of the trial (eight weeks) was relatively short. They reported a statistically significant group difference in improvement in repetitive behaviours ($p = 0.037$) and a large effect size (1.616). They acknowledged that this was a preliminary study. It should be noted that carbamazepine and sodium valproate/divalproex sodium are well-established mood-levelling drugs and it is consequently quite likely that any beneficial effect was through the mood-levelling properties rather than the antiepileptic effects. Topiramate is an antiepileptic drug with multiple modes of action; it is not surprising that it has been reported as showing both deleterious and beneficial effects on mood in various studies. Although the main role of antiepileptic drugs in children with autism and epilepsy is to control the seizures, in those who have mood disorders, choosing a medication that also has mood-levelling properties may be of benefit. Whether any additional benefit is derived from suppression of epileptiform discharges remains very much open to debate, as discussed elsewhere (Deonna and Roulet, 2006; Besag, 2009).

Both epilepsy and autism are associated with higher rates of coexisting psychiatric/behavioural problems. Viscidi et al. (2014) examined the association between epilepsy, autism spectrum disorder and maladaptive behaviours in 139 children. These were the children from the group of 2,645 subjects with autism spectrum disorder from the Simons Simplex Collection, of whom 139 additionally had epilepsy. The children with autism spectrum disorder who also had epilepsy had more autism symptoms and more maladaptive behaviours than those without epilepsy. However, they found that, after adjusting for IQ, only hyperactivity symptoms remained statistically significantly increased (13% higher) in the group of children with epilepsy. In the children who also had intellectual disability, the children with epilepsy had significantly more irritability (20% higher) and hyperactivity (24% higher) symptoms.

■ Future research

The area of genetics research has expanded to an extraordinary degree over recent years; this is true for genetics research into autism as it is into many other conditions. The results are complex but tantalising. Whether they will give precise guidance on management except in a small minority of cases remains to be seen.

Despite the disappointment expressed by Deonna and Roulet (2006), a large-scale prospective study in which 24-hour EEG, or at least an overnight/sleep EEG is performed in children as soon as any sign of regression becomes evident, might still be worthwhile. The evidence so far seems to indicate that such a study would identify only a very small number of children with epilepsy or epileptiform discharges, including electrical status epilepticus of slow-wave sleep, as the cause for the autism. However, if the clinical features of these children can be characterised, this could imply that, at least for this small subgroup, prompt and effective treatment might prevent further regression and allow some return of function.

Research into specific disorders in which autism is frequent, such as tuberous sclerosis complex, Rett syndrome and Fragile X syndrome, although interesting, have so far not yielded results that can be applied more generally to the management of autism. Nevertheless, continued research in these areas would appear to be worthwhile. An area of increasing interest is the role of neuronal antibodies in causing epilepsy and a number of psychiatric/psychological changes (Irani *et al.*, 2011; Vincent *et al.*, 2011). The role of neuronal antibodies in the complex relationships between epilepsy and autism is yet to be elucidated.

At present it must be concluded that, despite extensive research, there are still many unanswered questions regarding the relationships between epilepsy and autism.

References

Amiet, C., Gourfinkel-An, I., Bouzamondo, A., Tordjman, S., Baulac, M., Lechat, P., Mottron, L. & Cohen, D. 2008. Epilepsy in autism is associated with intellectual disability and gender: evidence from a meta-analysis. *Biological Psychiatry*, 64, 577-582.

Baird, G., Charman, T., Pickles, A., Chandler, S., Loucas, T., Meldrum, D., Carcani-Rathwell, I., Serkana, D. & Simonoff, E. 2008. Regression, developmental trajectory and associated problems in disorders in the autism spectrum: the SNAP study. *J.Autism Dev.Disord.*, 38, 1827-1836.

Baird, G., Robinson, R. O., Boyd, S. & Charman, T. 2006a. Sleep electroencephalograms in young children with autism with and without regression. *Developmental Medicine & Child Neurology*, 48, 604-608.

Baird, G., Simonoff, E., Pickles, A., Chandler, S., Loucas, T., Meldrum, D. & Charman, T. 2006b. Prevalence of disorders of the autism spectrum in a population cohort of children in South Thames: the Special Needs and Autism Project (SNAP). *Lancet*, 368, 210-215.

Berg, A. T., Plioplys, S. & Tuchman, R. 2011. Risk and correlates of autism spectrum disorder in children with epilepsy: a community-based study. *Journal of Child Neurology*, 26, 540-547.

Besag, F. M. C. 2009. The relationship between epilepsy and autism: a continuing debate. *Acta Paediatrica*, 98, 618-620.

Betancur, C. 2011. Etiological heterogeneity in autism spectrum disorders: more than 100 genetic and genomic disorders and still counting. *Brain Res.*, 1380, 42-77.

Bolton, P. F., Carcani-Rathwell, I., Hutton, J., Goode, S., Howlin, P. & Rutter, M. 2011. Epilepsy in autism: features and correlates. *The British Journal of Psychiatry*, 198, 289-294.

Brooks-Kayal, A. 2010. Epilepsy and autism spectrum disorders: are there common developmental mechanisms? *Brain and Development*, 32, 731-738.

Caraballo, R. H., Cejas, N., Chamorro, N., Kaltenmeier, M. C., Fortini, S. & Soprano, A. M. 2014. Landau-Kleffner syndrome: a study of 29 patients. *Seizure*, 23, 98-104.

Chez, M. G., Chang, M., Krasne, V., Coughlan, C., Kominsky, M. & Schwartz, A. 2006. Frequency of epileptiform EEG abnormalities in a sequential screening of autistic patients with no known clinical epilepsy from 1996 to 2005. *Epilepsy & Behavior*, 8, 267-271.

Childs, J. A. & Blair, J. L. 1997. Valproic acid treatment of epilepsy in autistic twins. *J.Neurosci.Nurs.*, 29, 244-248.

Clarke, D. F., Roberts, W., Daraksan, M., Dupuis, A., McCabe, J., Wood, H., Snead, O. C., III & Weiss, S. K. 2005. The prevalence of autistic spectrum disorder in children surveyed in a tertiary care epilepsy clinic. *Epilepsia*, 46, 1970-1977.

Cuccaro, M. L., Tuchman, R. F., Hamilton, K. L., Wright, H. H., Abramson, R. K., Haines, J. L., Gilbert, J. R. & Pericak-Vance, M. 2012. Exploring the relationship between autism spectrum disorder and epilepsy using latent class cluster analysis. *Journal of autism and developmental disorders*, 42, 1630-1641.

Danielsson, S., Gillberg, I. C., Billstedt, E., Gillberg, C. & Olsson, I. 2005. Epilepsy in young adults with autism: a prospective population-based follow-up study of 120 individuals diagnosed in childhood. *Epilepsia*, 46, 918-923.

Deonna, T. & Roulet, E. 2006. Autistic spectrum disorder: evaluating a possible contributing or causal role of epilepsy. *Epilepsia*, 47 Suppl 2, 79-82.

Gillberg, C. 1991. The treatment of epilepsy in autism. *J.Autism Dev.Disord.*, 21, 61-77.

Hardan, A. Y., Jou, R. J. & Handen, B. L. 2004. A retrospective assessment of topiramate in children and adolescents with pervasive developmental disorders. *J.Child Adolesc.Psychopharmacol.*, 14, 426-432.

Hollander, E., Soorya, L., Wasserman, S., Esposito, K., Chaplin, W. & Anagnostou, E. 2006. Divalproex sodium vs. placebo in the treatment of repetitive behaviours in autism spectrum disorder. *Int.J.Neuropsychopharmacol.*, 9, 209-213.

Irani, S. R., Bien, C. G. & Lang, B. 2011. Autoimmune epilepsies. *Current Opinion in Neurology*, 24, 146-153.

Jeavons, P. M. 1983. Non-epileptic attacks in childhood. In: CLIFFORD ROSE, F. (ed.) *Research Progress in Epilepsy*. London: Pitman.

Jokiranta, E., Sourander, A., Suominen, A., Timonen-Soivio, L., Brown, A. S. & Sillanpää, M. 2014. Epilepsy among children and adolescents with autism spectrum disorders: a population-based study. *Journal of Autism & Developmental Disorders*, 44, 2547-57.

Matsuo, M., Maeda, T., Sasaki, K., Ishii, K. & Hamasaki, Y. 2010. Frequent association of autism spectrum disorder in patients with childhood onset epilepsy. *Brain Dev.*, 32, 759-763.

Morrell, F., Whisler, W. W. & Bleck, T. P. 1989. Multiple subpial transection: a new approach to the surgical treatment of focal epilepsy. *Journal of Neurosurgery*, 70, 231-239.

Mouridsen, S. E., Rich, B. & Isager, T. 2011. A longitudinal study of epilepsy and other central nervous system diseases in individuals with and without a history of infantile autism. *Brain and Development*, 33, 361-366.

Nass, R. & Petrucha, D. 1990. Acquired aphasia with convulsive disorder: a pervasive developmental disorder variant. *J.Child Neurol.*, 5, 327-328.

Plioplys, A. V. 1994. Autism: electroencephalogram abnormalities and clinical improvement with valproic acid. *Arch.Pediatr.Adolesc.Med.*, 148, 220-222.

Robinson, S. J. 2012. Childhood epilepsy and autism spectrum disorders: psychiatric problems, phenotypic expression, and anticonvulsants. *Neuropsychol.Rev.*, 22, 271-279.

Roulet-Perez, E., Davidoff, V., Despland, P. A. & Deonna, T. 1993. Mental and behavioural deterioration of children with epilepsy and CSWS: acquired epileptic frontal syndrome. *Developmental Medicine & Child Neurology*, 35, 661-674.

Sillanpää, M. 1992. Epilepsy in children: prevalence, disability, and handicap. *Epilepsia*, 33, 444-449.

Spence, S. J. & Schneider, M. T. 2009. The role of epilepsy and epileptiform EEGs in autism spectrum disorders. *Pediatric Research*, 65, 599-606.

Steffenburg, S., Gillberg, C. & Steffenburg, U. 1996. Psychiatric disorders in children and adolescents with mental retardation and active epilepsy. *Archives of Neurology*, 53, 904-912.

Steffenburg, U., Hagberg, G., Viggedal, G. & Kyllerman, M. 1995. Active epilepsy in mentally retarded children. I. Prevalence and additional neuro-impairments. *Acta Paediatrica*, 84, 1147-1152.

Tharp, B. R. 2004. Epileptic encephalopathies and their relationship to developmental disorders: do spikes cause autism? *Ment Retard Dev Disabil Res Rev*, 10, 132-4.

Tuchman, R. 2013. Autism and social cognition in epilepsy: implications for comprehensive epilepsy care. *Current Opinion in Neurology*, 26, 214-218.

Tuchman, R., Alessandri, M. & Cuccaro, M. 2010. Autism spectrum disorders and epilepsy: moving towards a comprehensive approach to treatment. *Brain Dev.*, 32, 719-730.

Tuchman, R. & Cuccaro, M. 2011. Epilepsy and autism: neurodevelopmental perspective. *Current Neurology and Neuroscience Reports*, 11, 428-434.

Tuchman, R. & Rapin, I. 2002. Epilepsy in autism. *Lancet Neurology*, 1, 352-358.

Turk, J., Bax, M., Williams, C., Amin, P., Eriksson, M. & Gillberg, C. 2009. Autism spectrum disorder in children with and without epilepsy: impact on social functioning and communication. *Acta Paediatr*, 98, 675-81.

Uldall, P., Alving, J., Hansen, L. K., Kibaek, M. & Buchholt, J. 2006. The misdiagnosis of epilepsy in children admitted to a tertiary epilepsy centre with paroxysmal events. *Archives of Disease in Childhood*, 91, 219-221.

Uvebrant, P. & Bauziene, R. 1994. Intractable epilepsy in children. The efficacy of lamotrigine treatment, including non-seizure-related benefits. *Neuropediatrics*, 25, 284-289.

Vincent, A., Bien, C. G., Irani, S. R. & Waters, P. 2011. Autoantibodies associated with diseases of the CNS: new developments and future challenges. *Lancet Neurol*, 10, 759-72.

Viscidi, E. W., Johnson, A. L., Spence, S. J., Buka, S. L., Morrow, E. M. & Triche, E. W. 2014. The association between epilepsy and autism symptoms and maladaptive behaviors in children with autism spectrum disorder. *Autism*, 18, 996-1006.

Woolfenden, S., Sarkozy, V., Ridley, G., Coory, M. & Williams, K. 2012. A systematic review of two outcomes in autism spectrum disorder – epilepsy and mortality. *Dev.Med.Child Neurol.*, 54, 306-312.

Anxiety, depression and childhood epilepsy

David W. Dunn, Frank Besag, Rochelle Caplan,
Albert Aldenkamp, Giuseppe Gobbi, Matti Sillanpää6

Abstract

Anxiety and depression are relatively common in children with epilepsy: anxiety has been reported in 15-36% and depression in 8-35% of patients. In some cases these conditions may be related specifically to the epilepsy or its treatment. For example, some antiepileptic drugs are known to be associated with depression in adults and are likely to have a similar effect in young people. Emotional reactions to the epilepsy, for example anxieties and social phobia related specifically to the seizures, might be expected and require appropriate management. However, there is a growing recognition of the bidirectional relationship between epilepsy and psychiatric disorders, including depression, largely based on adult data. Cognitive behavioural therapy and serotonin reuptake inhibitors are used for treatment of both anxiety and depression in children with epilepsy. There is a need for greater understanding of the causes of these conditions in young people and there is also a need for better evidence for optimal treatment.

Key words: anxiety, depression, antiepileptic drug, cognitive behavioural therapy, antidepressant

Children and adolescents with epilepsy have an increased risk of anxiety and depression in comparison to healthy controls (Davies et al., 2003; Berg et al., 2011; Russ et al., 2012; Reilly et al., 2014). The association between internalizing disorders and epilepsy may have an adverse effect on quality of life but data on optimal treatment of anxiety and depression in children with epilepsy is limited.

■ Search strategy

A search was made using Ovid Medline for articles using the following terms: (anxiety or depression) and epilepsy and (childhood or adolescence) until March 2015. In addition, the references in review articles were used to identify articles missed in the Medline search.

Epidemiology

An increased prevalence of anxiety and depression in children with epilepsy has been found in both clinic-based and population-based studies. A British epidemiological survey reported emotional problems in 16.7% of children with complicated epilepsy, 16% of children with uncomplicated epilepsy, 6.4% of those with diabetes mellitus and 4.2% of healthy controls (Davies et al., 2003). In a long-term follow-up of children with new-onset seizures seen approximately nine years after their first seizure, Berg et al. (2011) noted depression in 13% and anxiety in 5% of children. In a large nationwide survey from the United States, Russ et al. (2012) found anxiety in 17% of children with current epilepsy, 9% of children with past seizures and 3% of controls, and depression in 8% of those with current epilepsy, 7% of children with past seizures and 2% of controls. Reilly et al. (2014), in a community-based study of children 5-15 years of age attending schools in Sussex, UK, found rates of 13% for anxiety and 7% for depression, using DSM-IV-TR criteria. They also made the point that very few of these children, only 1% for both disorders, had been diagnosed before the study had been performed, suggesting that in many children with epilepsy, anxiety and depression may go undiagnosed.

The reported prevalence figures from samples obtained in epilepsy clinics are, as might be expected, higher than those from epidemiological surveys. Studies from clinics have reported a prevalence of depression of 20-29% (range 9.6-36.5%) of children with epilepsy (Ettinger et al., 1998; Thomé-Souza et al., 2004; Dunn et al., 2009; Roeder et al., 2009) and a prevalence of anxiety of 27-36% (16-48%) (Ettinger et al., 1998; Alwash et al., 2000; Jones et al., 2007; Dunn et al., 2009). The variation in prevalence is most likely due to differences in populations and measures. The lowest prevalence for depression and epilepsy, 9.6%, was found in children and adolescents 9-14 years of age that had normal ability to mild intellectual disability. The diagnosis of depression was based on a checklist using strict DSM-IV criteria completed by parents (Dunn et al., 2009). In comparison, the sample with a prevalence of depression of 36.4% consisted of children and adolescents 4-18 years of age. Approximately half of the sample had an IQ of less than 70 (Thomé-Souza et al., 2004). The study reporting a prevalence of depression of 36.5% had a predominantly African-American population aged 6-17 years. The diagnosis of depression was based on a 13-item self-report questionnaire (Roeder et al., 2009). For anxiety, the lowest prevalence figure in clinical samples, 16%, was reported in a study of patients 7-18 years of age whose parents completed a 37-item anxiety disorder questionnaire (Ettinger et al., 1998). The highest prevalence of 48% was from a study of adolescents and young adults aged 14-24 years recruited from an epilepsy clinic in Jordan. The diagnosis of anxiety was based on a clinical interview (Alwash et al., 2000). It seems likely that adolescents report more symptoms of anxiety and depression than parents observe. Caplan et al. carried out a series of studies on psychopathology in children with epilepsy, from clinics or from the community. In a study of 101 children with complex partial (dyscognitive) seizures and 102 controls, aged 5.1 to 16.9 years, Caplan et al. (2004) found a rate of affective/anxiety disorder of 14% in children with epilepsy compared to 3% in controls. In a further study, Caplan et al. (2005) included 100 children with complex partial (dyscognitive) seizures and 71 children with childhood absence epilepsy. They found that children with epilepsy were five times more likely to have anxiety or depression than controls and that anxiety was more often reported than depression. Jones et al. (2007) studied 53 children, aged 8-18 years, 31M, 22F, with new-onset epilepsy, defined as a diagnosis of epilepsy within the past 12 months, who had no other developmental disabilities (for example, developmental delay or autism) from paediatric neurology clinics in two large mid-western medical centres in the US. They were compared with age-matched and sex-matched first-degree cousins (where available). The rate of depressive disorder was 22.6% compared with 4%, $p = 0.01$, and the rate of anxiety disorder was 35.8% compared with 22%, $p < 0.05$. Caplan et al. (2008) studied 69 children with specifically absence epilepsy. They found a rate of anxiety/depression of 29%. Of the 20 subjects identified, 15 had an anxiety disorder, four had depression and one had both conditions.

■ Phenomenology of anxiety and depression in children with epilepsy

The symptoms of anxiety and depression seen in children and adolescents with epilepsy are similar to those found in peers without seizures (Plioplys, 2003). In comparison to adults, children and adolescents with depression may be more irritable and moody, and children with anxiety may be tearful, clinging, or have tantrums. In a study of children 6-16 years of age with childhood absence epilepsy, Vega et al. (2011) found that the most common symptoms of anxiety were worrying, nervousness and negativity, and of depression were tearfulness, sadness and becoming easily upset, all symptoms that would be expected in a child without epilepsy who was experiencing anxiety or depression.

Some symptoms may relate specifically to epilepsy. Brief episodes of anxiety or fear can occur as an aura in children with focal epileptiform discharges from the temporal lobe or, less often, from the frontal lobe (Chiesa et al., 2007). Children with epilepsy may have anxieties related to their seizures. Approximately one-third of children with new-onset seizures report worrying about having another seizure and about talking to others about their seizure condition (McNelis et al., 1998). It seems likely that having recurrent seizures would lead to separation anxiety or social phobia but the data is limited. One study, from two university-based epilepsy clinics, found separation anxiety in 6% of children with epilepsy and 3% of adolescents with epilepsy; social phobia was found in 2% of children and 5% of adolescents with epilepsy (Dunn et al., 2009). A second university-based clinical study found separation anxiety in 32% and social phobia in 24% of the children with epilepsy and anxiety (Jones et al., 2015). Prevalence was higher than the 3.5% prevalence of separation anxiety and 1% rate of social phobia reported in epidemiological surveys of children in the general population (Costello et al., 2003).

Ictal and postictal depression has been described in adults with epilepsy (Kanner et al., 2004) but seems to be less common in children and adolescents. Similarly, an interictal dysphoric disorder has been reported in adults (Mula et al., 2008) but descriptions of interictal dysphoric disorder in children are not available.

■ Causes of anxiety and depression in children with epilepsy

Several risk factors for anxiety and depression in childhood epilepsy have been identified. The prevalence of anxiety in patients with epilepsy seems to be similar in childhood compared to adolescence but depression is more common in adolescents than younger children with epilepsy (Reilly et al., 2011). The gender difference of increased prevalence of anxiety and depression in adolescent girls seen in psychiatric populations is inconsistent and much less pronounced in adolescents with epilepsy (Reilly et al., 2011; Jones et al.,

2015). The risk of anxiety and depression is increased in children with epilepsy and lower IQ, language delays or decreasing scores on neuropsychological assessment (Buelow et al., 2003; Caplan et al., 2005; Austin et al., 2010).

Specific epilepsy-related factors do not seem to be a major factor in the causation of anxiety or depression. Age of seizure onset and seizure type or syndrome have not been consistent risk factors for anxiety or depression (Plioplys, 2003; Ekinci et al., 2009; Reilly et al., 2011; Jones et al., 2015). Anxiety and depression are more common in those with persistent seizures than in children or adolescents with well-controlled epilepsy (Berg et al., 2011). Symptoms of depression may occur as an adverse effect of GABA-ergic antiepileptic drugs such as phenobarbital, tiagabine or vigabatrin and have been associated with levetiracetam, topiramate and zonisamide (Kanner and Dunn, 2004). Depression may also follow discontinuation of lamotrigine, valproate and oxcarbazepine (Ketter et al., 1994; Barry et al., 2008). Anxiety has been associated with felbamate, levetiracetam and zonisamide (Mula and Sander, 2007; Weintraub et al., 2007) Most of the data relating to depression and anxiety associated with antiepileptic drugs has been in adults and has yet to be confirmed in children and adolescents (also see paper by Aldenkamp et al. in this series). [[Please add reference in the list]]

The psychological response to illness may be a significant contributor to internalizing problems. Dunn et al. (1999) found that the adolescent attitude toward illness and external or unknown locus of control were predictors of depression. Wagner et al. (2009) showed that hopelessness was an important factor in the association of epilepsy with depression in children and adolescents. Similarly, the adverse effect of seizures on the family may contribute to anxiety and depression in the child with epilepsy. Limited emotional support, poor communication, inadequate support of child autonomy and maternal depression are family factors that have been associated with depression in children and adolescents with epilepsy (Dunn et al., 1999; Austin et al., 2004; Rodenburg et al., 2006; Ferro and Speechley, 2009). One recent study found that parents of children with a first seizure had elevated levels of anxiety whereas an increased prevalence of anxiety was seen in children and adolescents with chronic seizures, suggesting that anxiety is not immediately transferred from parent to child (Save-Pedebos et al., 2014).

There is emerging evidence that a common underlying condition may predispose children and adolescents to both epilepsy and anxiety or depression. Kanner (2005) has suggested that abnormalities in serotonin or norepinephrine neurotransmitters, or dysfunction in frontal or temporal lobes may be involved in the aetiology of both epilepsy and depression. Jones et al. (2015), using structural MRI found enlargement of the amygdala and thinner cortex in the prefrontal and orbitofrontal regions, similar to that found in patients with anxiety without epilepsy. Genetic studies have shown a sharing of genetic risk factors in psychiatric disorders (Cross-Disorder Group of the Psychiatric Genomics, 2013) and neurodevelopmental disorders (Girirajan et al., 2012).

The association between behavioural problems and epilepsy may be bi-directional. A population-based study from Iceland of patients that were 10 years of age and older who had unprovoked seizures found that depression was a risk factor for subsequent seizures (Hesdorffer et al., 2006), and a survey of hospitalized patients, 33.3% of whom were less than 15 years of age, found that anxiety and depression predicted subsequent seizures (Adelow et al., 2012). Hesdorffer et al. (2012) have shown a familial clustering of uncomplicated epilepsy and behavioural disorders. In contrast, there was no association between family history of unprovoked seizures and behavioural problems when the probands had complicated seizures. Jones et al. (2015) also found that anxiety and depression were common in family members of children with epilepsy and anxiety.

The management of children with epilepsy and anxiety and/or depression

Kanner (2013) and Mula (2013) have pointed out the limited systematic data for the treatment of depression and anxiety in adults with epilepsy. There are even fewer controlled trials for internalizing disorders in children with epilepsy. As a result, practitioners must base treatment on clinical reasoning and the results of treatment trials conducted with children experiencing anxiety and/or depression without epilepsy (see consensus statement by Barry et al., 2008).

Although suicidal ideation/plans appear to be common in children with epilepsy and are associated with depression and anxiety, suicidal acts appear to be rare. For example, in the study by Caplan et al. (2005) in children with complex partial (dyscognitive) seizures and absence epilepsy, there were high rates of affective and anxiety disorder diagnoses (33%) and suicidal ideation/plan (20%) but no suicidal acts.

A reasonable first step in treatment is the assessment for possible reversible causes of anxiety or depression. Recent additions or changes in AEDs should prompt review for possible psychiatric adverse effects of medications. Medication adherence should be assessed and seizure control reviewed with a goal of complete seizure control without unacceptable psychiatric or other adverse effects.

A second step in treatment is education of the child and family. The data to support psychosocial treatments is limited by small sample sizes and inadequate outcome measures (Wagner and Smith, 2006), but series studies have shown that educational programs increase knowledge of epilepsy, reduce parental anxiety and improve child sense of competence (Lewis et al., 1990; Lewis et al., 1991; Tieffenberg et al., 2000; Wohlrab et al., 2007).

Cognitive behavioural therapy (CBT) has been used successfully in children and adolescents with anxiety and depression. Although no controlled trials are available in children and adolescents with epilepsy and anxiety or depression, one group has shown CBT to be effective in preventing the onset of depression in adolescents with epilepsy. Martinovic et al. (2006) compared CBT to treatment as usual in 104 adolescents with epilepsy. At nine-month follow up, symptoms of depression decreased in the CBT group and depressive disorder developed only in adolescents in the control group. Two studies with small sample sizes, seven participants in Snead et al. (2004) and nine in Wagner et al. (2010), reported the efficacy of interventions utilizing psychoeducation and CBT techniques. Snead et al. (2004) were able to show a trend for improved quality of life but no statistically significant change in measures of anxiety or depression. Wagner et al. (2010) found improvement in knowledge and self-efficacy but no change in symptoms of depression. In a pilot study of CBT for children with epilepsy and anxiety, Blocher et al. (2013) reported reduction in symptoms of anxiety and depression at the end of the 12 weeks of therapy and at three-month follow up. A systematic review of randomized controlled trials of CBT and case series in people with epilepsy found evidence of effectiveness for reducing symptoms of depression in people, mostly adults, with epilepsy but limited effect on improving seizure control (Gandy et al., 2014).

In children and adolescents with moderate to severe anxiety and/or depression, psychotropic medication should be considered. No controlled trials are available for children with epilepsy and anxiety or depression. One open-label trial reported that fluoxetine and sertraline were effective and safe in children and adolescents with epilepsy and depression. The sample consisted of 36 patients 6-17 years of age. All 36 patients had improvement in symptoms of depression and only two patients had a worsening of seizures (Thomé-Souza et al., 2007).

Treatment trials of adults with epilepsy and anxiety or depression, and randomized controlled trials of medication for anxiety and depression in children without epilepsy can be used as a guide for best treatment options. The selective serotonin reuptake inhibitors (SSRIs) are the first-choice medications. In the US, fluoxetine, sertraline and fluvoxamine are approved for treating anxiety in children; fluoxetine is approved for children and adolescents and escitalopram for adolescents with depression. The SSRIs and the serotonin norepinephrine reuptake inhibitors (SNRIs) are used off-label for anxiety and depression in children and adolescents. The SSRIs and the SNRIs do not reduce seizure threshold and may even lessen the chance of seizures (Alper et al., 2007). Fluoxetine and fluvoxamine are inhibitors of cytochrome P450 enzymes and may cause elevations of phenytoin, carbamazepine and valproate levels. Phenobarbital, phenytoin, and carbamazepine also induce CYP enzymes and may lower the serum levels of SSRIs and SNRIs.

Pregabalin has been recommended as a first-choice treatment for generalized anxiety disorder in adults with epilepsy but no data exists for treatment of children with anxiety and epilepsy (Mula, 2013). The tricyclic antidepressants have not been effective in the treatment of childhood depression and have shown inconsistent effect in the treatment of childhood anxiety. The tricyclic antidepressants, in particular clomipramine, may lower seizure threshold and thus should be used cautiously if at all in children with epilepsy and anxiety or depression. Bupropion is an aminoketone antidepressant that may lower seizure threshold at higher doses and is not recommended for children with epilepsy. There are no convincing data to recommend the use of benzodiazepines or buspirone in children with epilepsy and anxiety.

Conclusions and recommendations for future research

Anxiety and depression are common in children and adolescents with epilepsy, affecting one-quarter to one-third of patients. Multiple epilepsy-related, psychological and genetic-familial factors have been implicated in causing anxiety and depression in patients with epilepsy. Understanding of the genetic and biological factors underlying the combination of epilepsy and emotional problems is developing rapidly and may lead to new therapeutic options. Currently, serotonin reuptake inhibitors and cognitive behavioural therapy are accepted treatments, although studies in populations with epilepsy are limited. Adequate studies of both behavioural and pharmacological treatments for anxiety and depression in children and adolescents with epilepsy are missing and are clearly needed to enhance quality of life in these patients.

References

Adelow C, Andersson T, Ahlbom A, Tomson T. Hospitalization for psychiatric disorders before and after onset of unprovoked seizures/epilepsy. *Neurology* 2012; 78(6): 396-401.

Alper K, Schwartz KA, Kolts RL, Khan A. Seizure incidence in psychopharmacological clinical trials: an analysis of Food and Drug Administration (FDA) summary basis of approval reports. *Biological Psychiatry* 2007; 62(4): 345-354.

Alwash RH, Hussein MJ, Matloub FF. Symptoms of anxiety and depression among adolescents with seizures in Irbid, Northern Jordan. *Seizure* 2000; 9(6): 412-6.

Austin JK, Dunn DW, Johnson CS, Perkins SM. Behavioral issues involving children and adolescents with epilepsy and the impact of their families: recent research data. *Epilepsy Behav* 2004; 5 Suppl 3: S33-41.

Austin JK, Perkins SM, Johnson CS, Fastenau PS, Byars AW, deGrauw TJ, et al. Self-esteem and symptoms of depression in children with seizures: relationships with neuropsychological functioning and family variables over time. *Epilepsia* 2010; 51(10): 2074-83.

Barry JJ, Ettinger AB, Friel P, Gilliam FG, Harden CL, Hermann B, et al. Consensus statement: the evaluation and treatment of people with epilepsy and affective disorders. *Epilepsy Behav* 2008; 13 Suppl 1: S1-29.

Berg AT, Caplan R, Hesdorffer DC. Psychiatric and neurodevelopmental disorders in childhood-onset epilepsy. *Epilepsy Behav* 2011; 20(3): 550-5.

Blocher JB, Fujikawa M, Sung C, Jackson DC, Jones JE. Computer-assisted cognitive behavioral therapy for children with epilepsy and anxiety: a pilot study. *Epilepsy Behav* 2013; 27(1): 70-6.

Buelow JM, Austin JK, Perkins SM, Shen J, Dunn DW, Fastenau PS. Behavior and mental health problems in children with epilepsy and low IQ. *Dev Med Child Neurol* 2003; 45(10): 683-92.

Caplan R, Siddarth P, Gurbani S, Hanson R, Sankar R, Shields WD. Depression and anxiety disorders in pediatric epilepsy. *Epilepsia* 2005; 46(5): 720-30.

Caplan R, Siddarth P, Gurbani S, Ott D, Sankar R, Shields WD. Psychopathology and pediatric complex partial seizures: seizure-related, cognitive, and linguistic variables. *Epilepsia* 2004; 45(10): 1273-1281.

Caplan R, Siddarth P, Stahl L, Lanphier E, Vona P, Gurbani S, et al. Childhood absence epilepsy: behavioral, cognitive, and linguistic comorbidities. *Epilepsia* 2008; 49(11): 1838-1846.

Chiesa V, Gardella E, Tassi L, Canger R, Lo Russo G, Piazzini A, et al. Age-related gender differences in reporting ictal fear: analysis of case histories and review of the literature. *Epilepsia* 2007; 48(12): 2361-4.

Costello EJ, Mustillo S, Erkanli A, Keeler G, Angold A. Prevalence and development of psychiatric disorders in childhood and adolescence. *Arch Gen Psychiatry* 2003; 60(8): 837-44.

Cross-Disorder Group of the Psychiatric Genomics C. Identification of risk loci with shared effects on five major psychiatric disorders: a genome-wide analysis. *Lancet* 2013; 381(9875): 1371-9.

Davies S, Heyman I, Goodman R. A population survey of mental health problems in children with epilepsy. *Developmental Medicine & Child Neurology* 2003; 45(5): 292-295.

Dunn DW, Austin JK, Huster GA. Symptoms of depression in adolescents with epilepsy. *Journal of the American Academy of Child & Adolescent Psychiatry* 1999; 38(9): 1132-1138.

Dunn DW, Austin JK, Perkins SM. Prevalence of psychopathology in childhood epilepsy: categorical and dimensional measures. *Developmental Medicine & Child Neurology* 2009; 51(5): 364-372.

Ekinci O, Titus JB, Rodopman AA, Berkem M, Trevathan E. Depression and anxiety in children and adolescents with epilepsy: prevalence, risk factors, and treatment. *Epilepsy Behav* 2009; 14(1): 8-18.

Ettinger AB, Weisbrot DM, Nolan EE, Gadow KD, Vitale SA, Andriola MR, et al. Symptoms of depression and anxiety in pediatric epilepsy patients. *Epilepsia* 1998; 39(6): 595-9.

Ferro MA, Speechley KN. Depressive symptoms among mothers of children with epilepsy: a review of prevalence, associated factors, and impact on children. *Epilepsia* 2009; 50(11): 2344-54.

Gandy M, Sharpe L, Nicholson Perry K, Thayer Z, Miller L, Boserio J, et al. Cognitive behaviour therapy to improve mood in people with epilepsy: a randomised controlled trial. *Cogn Behav Ther* 2014; 43(2): 153-66.

Girirajan S, Rosenfeld JA, Coe BP, Parikh S, Friedman N, Goldstein A, et al. Phenotypic heterogeneity of genomic disorders and rare copy-number variants. *N Engl J Med* 2012; 367(14): 1321-31.

Hesdorffer DC, Caplan R, Berg AT. Familial clustering of epilepsy and behavioral disorders: evidence for a shared genetic basis. *Epilepsia* 2012; 53(2): 301-307.

Hesdorffer DC, Hauser WA, Olafsson E, Ludvigsson P, Kjartansson O. Depression and suicide attempt as risk factors for incident unprovoked seizures. *Ann Neurol* 2006; 59(1): 35-41.

Jones JE, Jackson DC, Chambers KL, Dabbs K, Hsu DA, Stafstrom CE, et al. Children with epilepsy and anxiety: Subcortical and cortical differences. *Epilepsia* 2015; 56(2): 283-90.

Jones JE, Watson R, Sheth R, Caplan R, Koehn M, Seidenberg M, et al. Psychiatric comorbidity in children with new onset epilepsy. *Dev.Med.Child Neurol.* 2007; 49(7): 493-497.

Kanner AM. The treatment of depressive disorders in epilepsy: what all neurologists should know. *Epilepsia* 2013; 54 Suppl 1: 3-12.

Kanner AM. Depression in epilepsy: a neurobiologic perspective. *Epilepsy Curr* 2005; 5(1): 21-7.

Kanner AM, Dunn DW. Diagnosis and management of depression and psychosis in children and adolescents with epilepsy. *Journal of Child Neurology* 2004; 19: Suppl-72.

Kanner AM, Soto A, Gross-Kanner H. Prevalence and clinical characteristics of postictal psychiatric symptoms in partial epilepsy. *Neurology* 2004; 62(5): 708-13.

Ketter TA, Malow BA, Flamini R, White SR, Post RM, Theodore WH. Anticonvulsant withdrawal-emergent psychopathology. *Neurology* 1994; 44(1): 55-61.

Lewis MA, Hatton CL, Salas I, Leake B, Chiofalo N. Impact of the Children's Epilepsy Program on parents. *Epilepsia* 1991; 32(3): 365-74.

Lewis MA, Salas I, de la Sota A, Chiofalo N, Leake B. Randomized trial of a program to enhance the competencies of children with epilepsy. *Epilepsia* 1990; 31(1): 101-9.

Martinovic Z, Simonovic P, Djokic R. Preventing depression in adolescents with epilepsy. *Epilepsy Behav* 2006; 9(4): 619-24.

McNelis A, Musick B, Austin J, Dunn D, Creasy K. Psychosocial care needs of children with new-onset seizures. 2. *J Neurosci Nurs* 1998; 30(3): 161-5.

Mula M. Treatment of anxiety disorders in epilepsy: an evidence-based approach. *Epilepsia* 2013; 54 Suppl 1: 13-8.

Mula M, Jauch R, Cavanna A, Collimedaglia L, Barbagli D, Gaus V, et al. Clinical and psychopathological definition of the interictal dysphoric disorder of epilepsy. *Epilepsia* 2008; 49(4): 650-6.

Mula M, Sander JW. Negative effects of antiepileptic drugs on mood in patients with epilepsy. *Drug Saf* 2007; 30(7): 555-67.

Plioplys S. Depression in children and adolescents with epilepsy. *Epilepsy Behav* 2003; 4 Suppl 3: S39-45.

Reilly C, Agnew R, Neville BG. Depression and anxiety in childhood epilepsy: a review. *Seizure* 2011; 20(8): 589-597.

Reilly C, Atkinson P, Das KB, Chin RF, Aylett SE, Burch V, et al. Neurobehavioral comorbidities in children with active epilepsy: a population-based study. *Pediatrics* 2014; 133(6): e1586-93.

Rodenburg R, Marie Meijer A, Dekovic M, Aldenkamp AP. Family predictors of psychopathology in children with epilepsy. *Epilepsia* 2006; 47(3): 601-14.

Roeder R, Roeder K, Asano E, Chugani HT. Depression and mental health help-seeking behaviors in a predominantly African American population of children and adolescents with epilepsy. *Epilepsia* 2009; 50(8): 1943-52.

Russ SA, Larson K, Halfon N. A national profile of childhood epilepsy and seizure disorder. *Pediatrics* 2012; 129(2): 256-264.

Save-Pedebos J, Bellavoine V, Goujon E, Danse M, Merdariu D, Dournaud P, *et al*. Difference in anxiety symptoms between children and their parents facing a first seizure or epilepsy. *Epilepsy Behav* 2014; 31: 97-101.

Snead K, Ackerson J, Bailey K, Schmitt MM, Madan-Swain A, Martin RC. Taking charge of epilepsy: the development of a structured psychoeducational group intervention for adolescents with epilepsy and their parents. *Epilepsy Behav* 2004; 5(4): 547-56.

Thomé-Souza S, Kuczynski E, Assumpção Jr F, Rzezak P, Fuentes D, Fiore L, *et al*. Which factors may play a pivotal role on determining the type of psychiatric disorder in children and adolescents with epilepsy? *Epilepsy & Behavior* 2004; 5(6): 988-994.

Thomé-Souza S, Kuczynski E, Valente K. Sertraline and fluoxetine: safe treatments for children and adolescents with epilepsy and depression. *Epilepsy Behav* 2007; 10(3): 417-25.

Tieffenberg JA, Wood EI, Alonso A, Tossutti MS, Vicente MF. A randomized field trial of ACINDES: a child-centered training model for children with chronic illnesses (asthma and epilepsy). *J Urban Health* 2000; 77(2): 280-97.

Vega C, Guo J, Killory B, Danielson N, Vestal M, Berman R, *et al*. Symptoms of anxiety and depression in childhood absence epilepsy. *Epilepsia* 2011; 52(8): e70-4.

Wagner JL, Smith G. Psychosocial intervention in pediatric epilepsy: a critique of the literature. *Epilepsy Behav* 2006; 8(1): 39-49.

Wagner JL, Smith G, Ferguson P, van Bakergem K, Hrisko S. Pilot study of an integrated cognitive-behavioral and self-management intervention for youth with epilepsy and caregivers: Coping Openly and Personally with Epilepsy (COPE). *Epilepsy Behav* 2010; 18(3): 280-5.

Wagner JL, Smith G, Ferguson PL, Horton S, Wilson E. A hopelessness model of depressive symptoms in youth with epilepsy. *J Pediatr Psychol* 2009; 34(1): 89-96.

Weintraub D, Buchsbaum R, Resor SR, Jr., Hirsch LJ. Psychiatric and behavioral side effects of the newer antiepileptic drugs in adults with epilepsy. *Epilepsy Behav* 2007; 10(1): 105-10.

Wohlrab GC, Rinnert S, Bettendorf U, Fischbach H, Heinen G, Klein P, *et al*. famoses: a modular educational program for children with epilepsy and their parents. *Epilepsy Behav* 2007; 10(1): 44-8.

Epilepsy and psychosis in children and teenagers

Frank Besag, Rochelle Caplan, Albert Aldenkamp, David W. Dunn, Giuseppe Gobbi, Matti Sillanpää

Abstract

Psychosis related to epilepsy or antiepileptic treatment can occur in teenagers and very rarely in children. Postictal, interictal and antiepileptic-drug-induced psychosis have all been reported in young people. Whether ictal psychosis occurs in this age group remains open to debate. Neuronal antibody encephalitis such as anti-NMDA receptor encephalitis can present with seizures and psychosis, both of which can resolve with prompt, appropriate immunotherapy. In addition, there have been several reports in which the terms psychosis or psychotic features have been used loosely to describe behavioural disturbance in children with epilepsy; in these cases there have apparently been no diagnostic features of psychosis, implying that these terms should not have been used. The management of epilepsy-related psychosis in young people is similar to that in adults. Antipsychotic medication should not be withheld if it is needed on clinical grounds. If the psychosis has been induced by antiepileptic medication then a medication review is necessary.

Key words: psychosis, postictal, interictal, antiepileptic drug, schizophrenia, affective

Clark *et al.* (2012) carried out a population study of children born in Helsinki between 1947 and 1990, which demonstrated a shared risk between epilepsy and psychosis. The total sample was of 9653 families with 23,404 offspring. Those with epilepsy had a 5.5-fold increased risk of having a broadly-defined psychotic disorder and almost an 8.5 fold increase in the risk of having schizophrenia. There was clustering of the association between epilepsy and psychosis in families, suggesting a strong genetic link. Individuals with a parental history of epilepsy had a twofold increase in risk of developing psychosis; individuals with a parental history of psychosis had a 2.7 fold increase in the risk of having generalised epilepsy, indicating a reciprocal relationship between the two conditions.

Most of the reports of psychosis associated with epilepsy are in adults. Lax Pericall and Taylor (2010) identified 17 individuals in a retrospective study of young people under 19 years of age with epilepsy who developed psychosis. Compared with young people who had psychosis without epilepsy, those with epilepsy had a higher rate of neuropsychological problems such as intellectual impairment or autism. In contrast to the situation for adults, the psychosis was not specifically associated with temporal lobe epilepsy or mesial temporal sclerosis. The individuals had a variety of seizure types and structural abnormalities.

Although many papers report psychosis or "psychotic features" in children with epilepsy, in a large proportion of these reports no formal diagnosis has been made and the term is being used loosely to describe behaviour that cannot easily be explained; no evidence for features such as hallucinations, delusions or thought disorder are provided. However, psychosis does occur in young people with epilepsy and appears to have the same causes as psychosis in adults. Psychosis is rare in children (as opposed to teenagers) in the general population and this also holds true for children with epilepsy. Psychosis in teenagers with epilepsy can be postictal, interictal, antiepileptic-drug-induced or post-surgery. Whether ictal psychosis occurs in teenagers remains open to debate. To these categories should, of course, be added psychosis that appears to be unrelated either to the epilepsy or its treatment; however, there are difficulties in distinguishing this category clearly from others. First, it may be difficult to distinguish it from the classical so-called "interictal psychosis". Second, as already stated, there appear to be underlying genetic links between epilepsy and psychiatric disorder, particularly schizophrenia; there is good epidemiological evidence for a bidirectional relationship between epilepsy and psychosis (Wotton and Goldacre, 2012; Adelow et al., 2012; Qin et al., 2005; Clarke et al., 2012). The concepts of "alternative psychosis" or "reciprocal psychosis" and "forced normalisation" will also be discussed in what follows. The various causes and categories of psychosis in children and teenagers with epilepsy will be considered in detail.

■ Search strategy

The Medline/PubMed database was searched from inception until the end of March 2015 using the search terms: epilep$ and (child$ or pediat$ or adolescen$) and (psychosis or psychotic or schizopren$). Abstracts of likely relevance to the topic were examined to select papers for final detailed review. Reference lists of included papers were searched for any further relevant studies.

■ Ictal psychosis

The phenomenon of psychotic features that are a direct effect of the seizure and last only for the duration of the seizure activity has been described by Kanemoto et al. (2012) in adults but there appear to be few, if any, reports in teenagers. In the experience of the authors, some children with frequent absence seizures have such fragmented thought processes that their speech might be interpreted as resembling the formal thought disorder of schizophrenia. However, this should not be interpreted as psychosis; it is potentially treatable epilepsy. It is not accompanied by hallucinations or delusions.

Interictal psychosis

There is confusion surrounding this term. Strictly speaking, it should refer to psychosis that occurs between seizures but in no clear time relation to them (in contrast to postictal psychosis, in which there is a clear time relationship to the seizures – see later). However, in the literature the term "interictal psychosis" is frequently used to describe psychosis with onset several years after the patient has become seizure free, as described in the classical paper by Slater and Beard (1995) in adults. Strictly speaking, this phenomenon might better be termed "post-epilepsy psychosis", since the onset is not until after the patient has been seizure free for many years. However, the term interictal psychosis appears to have become well-established in this context and it would not be practicable to change the terminology at this stage. True interictal psychosis, that is psychosis between the seizures but having no clear time relationship to them, can also occur, but is infrequent (Caplan et al., 1991; Caplan et al., 2004).

Adachi et al. (2012), in their study of 155 patients with 320 interictal psychosis episodes, noted that the age range was 14-66 years, implying that some of the patients were teenagers, although the mean age of onset was 30.9 years. The interval between the onset of epilepsy and the first interictal psychosis episode was 18.3 years (0-55 years). Although this was not a population study, the pattern reported is consistent with clinical experience: interictal psychosis is much more commonly reported in adults but can sometimes occur in teenagers, even in the earlier teenage years.

What is the relationship between interictal psychosis and reciprocal (alternative) psychosis? The terms "reciprocal psychosis" and "alternative psychosis" can be used interchangeably. Again, there is some confusion amongst practitioners about terminology, particularly between reciprocal psychosis and forced normalisation. Reciprocal psychosis is the phenomenon of "seizures better, psychosis worse" and "seizures worse, psychosis better (resolved)". This is a purely clinical phenomenon and does not require any EEG investigation to confirm it. In contrast, the phenomenon of "forced normalisation" can only be diagnosed with the aid of the EEG. It refers to the situation of "EEG better, psychosis worse" and "EEG worse, psychosis better (resolved)". The phenomena of reciprocal psychosis and forced normalisation are clearly related but they are not identical. To add to the confusion, sometimes the EEG can appear to be worse (in terms of epileptiform discharges), not better when the psychosis is worse. Some might argue that this could represent "ictal psychosis" but with no other obvious seizure-related clinical phenomena, it would be difficult to apply this diagnosis. A further difficulty arises when psychosis appears after the prescription of an antiepileptic drug. Has the psychosis arisen because the seizures have suddenly been controlled, in which case it could be viewed as a reciprocal psychosis, or is this an antiepileptic-drug-induced psychosis, that has arisen because a specific antiepileptic drug with psychosis as an adverse effect has been prescribed? Psychosis precipitated by vigabatrin (Cánovas Martínez et al., 1995), topiramate (Reith et al., 2003) or levetiracetam (Kossoff et al., 2001) can occur in young people. There was a suspicion, soon after some of the newer antiepileptic drugs became available, that slow escalation when the drug was first prescribed would be associated with a lower rate of psychiatric adverse events. This was subsequently shown to be the case in adult practice by Mula et al. (2003). Does this imply that some of the cases of psychosis attributed to antiepileptic drugs were actually cases of reciprocal psychosis that resulted from the seizures being controlled too rapidly or were these cases of a genuine drug-induced psychosis that was independent of seizure control? Was the decrease in the likelihood of psychosis by slow introduction of the antiepileptic medication simply an example of what is seen with many other adverse effects of antiepileptic drugs, namely that following the rule of "start low, go slow" greatly reduces the frequency of adverse effects? It is not always easy to distinguish between these two situations of alternative psychosis and drug-induced psychosis. The fact that certain antiepileptic drugs are particularly associated with psychosis might be taken as indicating that it is, indeed, the drugs themselves that are responsible but this would only be a sound argument if it could be shown that other antiepileptic drugs that were equally rapid and effective in controlling seizures did not precipitate psychosis to the same extent. Such data are difficult to collect; the numbers are very small when stratified for possible confounding factors such as type of epilepsy, concomitant medication, personal or family history of psychiatric disorder (Qin et al., 2005) and various other issues. In addition, interictal psychosis in which the EEG is worse, not better, can occur in children and teenagers with epilepsy (Caplan et al., 1991). It appears that drug-induced psychosis can also occur in young people, as described later, although the debate about whether some of these cases represent "alternative psychosis" will remain.

Although most of the psychosis cases that are drawn to the attention of the clinician are schizophreniform psychoses, manic psychosis can also occur in teenagers with a history of epilepsy. In the experience of the authors, this has been the so-called "interictal psychosis", which is not truly interictal but follows many years after the seizures have ceased to occur. This type of manic psychosis can be recurrent. It can respond well to sodium valproate, prescribed not as an antiepileptic drug but as a mood-levelling drug, in the experience of at least one of the current authors.

■ Postictal psychosis

This phenomenon has been well described in adults (Kanemoto et al., 1996) but can also occur in teenagers. The usual situation is that a teenager with epilepsy but with no previous history of psychosis has a cluster of seizures, after which he/she has delusions or hallucinations. The situation for teenagers is less well documented than it is for adults but the current authors have had experience of cases as young as 14 years of age. The adult data indicate that the individual may not develop the psychosis immediately following the cluster of seizures; it can develop after an interval of up to three days or sometimes longer. Whether this "lucid interval" described for adults can also occur for teenagers remains unclear. Postictal psychosis is generally thought to be self-limiting and, if not severe or distressing either to the individual or family, might not warrant treatment. In practice, short-term treatment may be indicated. An atypical antipsychotic drug such as risperidone is usually chosen. This may be continued for a few weeks and then slowly decreased, monitoring the patient for a re-emergence of the psychotic symptoms. Postictal psychosis can be recurrent and it is important to warn the family of this possibility so as to ensure prompt treatment on future occasions. They should be informed of the need to monitor for possible signs of the psychosis after subsequent clusters of seizures; the psychiatrist should agree an arrangement with the family to ensure prompt re-assessment, with treatment if required. This will reduce the duration and probably the extent of any distress experienced by the individual and family.

■ Antiepileptic drug-induced psychosis

Both topiramate and vigabatrin can induce psychosis in teenagers with epilepsy. The current authors have seen examples of both these situations in their own teenage patients.

There have been occasional reports of psychosis precipitated by other antiepileptic drugs. Youroukos et al. (2003) reported the case of a 12-year-old girl with idiopathic partial seizures with secondary generalisation who developed psychosis 10 days after levetiracetam was added to sodium valproate. Kossoff et al. (2001) published four case reports of psychosis developing after the commencement of levetiracetam; one of the four was a child of 9 years of age and the other three were teenagers. The psychosis manifested as hallucinations and/or delusions. After the levetiracetam was discontinued the psychosis resolved promptly. Hirose et al. (2003) reported a single case of apparent reciprocal psychosis (described by the authors as "forced normalisation") with severe psychotic features after zonisamide was commenced in a 5-year-old girl with previously uncontrolled seizures that became completely controlled with this drug. Her mental state did not resolve when the zonisamide was discontinued. She improved gradually following the prescription of fluvoxamine but the seizures also reappeared.

As already discussed, the risk factors that apply to adults probably also apply to teenagers. Psychosis following the prescription of at least some antiepileptic drugs will probably be much less common now that the importance of starting at a low dose and escalating the dose slowly have been emphasised (Mula et al., 2003). Again, drawing on the adult data, it would be wise to ensure careful monitoring of any teenager who has a personal or family history of psychiatric disorder. In such cases the starting dose and escalation rate should be particularly slow and specific enquiry should be made about abnormal phenomena such as delusions or hallucinations during the early phase of treatment. There are no firm guidelines for how to manage this situation if abnormal mental phenomena develop after the prescription of antiepileptic medication. Some might stop the antiepileptic medication altogether, provided the risk of a serious seizure exacerbation is not too great, whereas others would try a dose reduction, possibly followed by even slower re-escalation. In practice, when psychosis develops after the introduction of a drug, the individual or family, recognising the association between the drug and the psychosis, is highly likely to request that it be replaced by another antiepileptic drug. Continuing the suspect antiepileptic drug and treating the drug-induced psychosis with neuroleptic medication would not usually be recommended. The general principle of avoiding treatment of the adverse effects of one drug by prescribing another drug, if at all possible, should apply. However, each case must be managed individually.

Psychosis following epilepsy surgery

Although psychosis is reported following temporal lobectomy in adults (see Macrodimitris, 2011, for a review) there appears to be a dearth of studies in children and teenagers. The occasional occurrence of post-temporal lobectomy psychotic features in teenagers seems to follow the pattern described in some adult series: onset and persistence in the early weeks after surgery, followed by resolution in the longer term. This is in keeping with the experience of the current authors. However, there is a lack of data to confirm whether this anecdotal information is a true reflection of the likely sequence of events. Krayem et al. (2014) described a single case report of an 11-year-old girl who required repeated admission from 9 years of age for psychosis after right temporal resection at 3 years of age for an astrocytoma but this case was complicated by recurrence of the tumour.

■ Neuronal antibodies

In recent years there has been an increasing recognition of the importance of neuronal antibodies presenting with seizures, psychosis and other clinical features. These are well described in landmark papers by Vincent, Dalmau and others (Vincent et al., 2011; Dalmau et al., 2008). In particular, anti-NMDA antibody encephalitis can present with seizures and psychosis. The series of a hundred cases of this condition published by Dalmau et al. (2008) included both children and adults. A recent case report (Slettedal et al., 2012) described a school-age girl (exact age not stated) who had seizures affecting the left side of her face and left arm, together with a psychiatric presentation of anxiety, aggressive behaviour and delusions. Her condition worsened, despite treatment with carbamazepine and chlorpromazine. She did not respond to steroids or intravenous immunoglobulin but there was an immediate improvement followed by gradual recovery when she was treated with plasmapheresis in the ninth week of the illness, followed by gradual recovery. The authors summarised the five phases of anti-NMDA receptor encephalitis: the prodromal phase, the psychotic phase, the non-responsive phase, the hyperkinetic phase and gradual recovery. The importance of recognising neuronal antibody encephalitis and treating it promptly with appropriate immunotherapy cannot be over-emphasised. This is an extraordinary situation in which both the epilepsy and psychosis can be cured with medical treatment.

■ Conclusions

Epilepsy-associated psychosis of various types can occur in teenagers and very rarely in children. It is quite clear that interictal and postictal psychosis occur. It is less clear whether ictal psychosis can occur in children or teenagers. Neuronal antibody encephalitis such as anti-NMDA receptor encephalitis can present with seizures and psychosis; prompt treatment with appropriate immunotherapy can be curative in such cases. Psychosis in association with the prescription of some antiepileptic drugs can also occur in children and teenagers. Although the data on teenagers with psychosis is somewhat limited, there seems every reason to recommend starting at low doses and escalating the dose slowly when antiepileptic drugs that have a documented association with psychosis, such as vigabatrin and topiramate, are being prescribed. If the psychosis is drug-induced, a review of the antiepileptic medication is indicated. If the psychosis is not drug-induced and requires neuroleptic treatment, this should not normally be withheld on the basis of possible seizure exacerbation. For most antipsychotic drugs, the risk of seizure exacerbation is very low, with the exception of clozapine, which would not be prescribed as first-line antipsychotic medication in any case. For postictal psychosis, the antipsychotic treatment can be withdrawn slowly when the psychotic features have resolved but further antipsychotic treatment might be required for future episodes of postictal psychosis. The uncommon situation of manic psychosis can sometimes be treated satisfactorily with mood-levelling antiepileptic medication, such as sodium valproate. It is important to emphasise that antipsychotic treatment should not be withheld if the psychosis is associated with significant risk or if it is causing distress to the individual and/or their family. Prompt, effective treatment is likely to decrease the duration and degree of such distress greatly.

References

Adachi N, Akanuma N, Ito M, Okazaki M, Kato M, Onuma T. Interictal psychotic episodes in epilepsy: duration and associated clinical factors. *Epilepsia* 2012; 53(6): 1088-94.

Adelow C, Andersson T, Ahlbom A, Tomson T. Hospitalization for psychiatric disorders before and after onset of unprovoked seizures/epilepsy. *Neurology* 2012; 78(6): 396-401.

Cánovas Martínez A, Ordovás Baines J, Beltrán Marqués M, Escrivá Aparisi A, Delgado Cordón F. Vigabatrin-associated reversible acute psychosis in a child. *Annals of Pharmacotherapy* 1995; 29(11): 1115-1117.

Caplan R, Shields WD, Mori L, Yudovin S. Middle childhood onset of interictal psychosis. *J.Am.Acad.Child Adolesc.Psychiatry* 1991; 30(6): 893-896.

Caplan R, Siddarth P, Gurbani S, Ott D, Sankar R, Shields WD. Psychopathology and pediatric complex partial seizures: seizure-related, cognitive, and linguistic variables. *Epilepsia* 2004; 45(10): 1273-1281.

Clarke MC, Tanskanen A, Huttunen MO, Clancy M, Cotter DR, Cannon M. Evidence for shared susceptibility to epilepsy and psychosis: a population-based family study. *Biol Psychiatry* 2012; 71(9): 836-9.

Dalmau J, Gleichman AJ, Hughes EG, Rossi JE, Peng X, Lai M, *et al*. Anti-NMDA-receptor encephalitis: case series and analysis of the effects of antibodies. *Lancet Neurol* 2008; 7(12): 1091-8.

Hirose M, Yokoyama H, Haginoya K, Iinuma K. A five-year-old girl with epilepsy showing forced normalization due to zonisamide. *No To Hattatsu* 2003; 35(3): 259-263.

Kanemoto K, Kawasaki J, Kawai I. Postictal psychosis: a comparison with acute interictal and chronic psychoses. *Epilepsia* 1996; 37(6): 551-6.

Kanemoto K, Tadokoro Y, Oshima T. Psychotic illness in patients with epilepsy. *Ther.Adv.Neurol.Disord.* 2012; 5(6): 321-334.

Kossoff EH, Bergey GK, Freeman JM, Vining EP. Levetiracetam psychosis in children with epilepsy. *Epilepsia* 2001; 42(12): 1611-1613.

Krayem BH, Dunn NR, Swift RG. Psychosis after right temporal lobe tumor resection and recurrence. *J Neuropsychiatry Clin Neurosci* 2014; 26(1): E47.

Lax Pericall MT, Taylor E. Psychosis and epilepsy in young people. *Epilepsy Behav* 2010; 18(4): 450-4.

Macrodimitris S, Sherman EM, Forde S, Tellez-Zenteno JF, Metcalfe A, Hernandez-Ronquillo L, *et al*. Psychiatric outcomes of epilepsy surgery: a systematic review. *Epilepsia* 2011; 52(5): 880-890.

Mula M, Trimble MR, Lhatoo SD, Sander JW. Topiramate and psychiatric adverse events in patients with epilepsy. *Epilepsia* 2003; 44(5): 659-663.

Qin P, Xu H, Laursen TM, Vestergaard M, Mortensen PB. Risk for schizophrenia and schizophrenia-like psychosis among patients with epilepsy: population based cohort study. *BMJ* 2005; 331(7507): 23.

Reith D, Burke C, Appleton DB, Wallace G, Pelekanos J. Tolerability of topiramate in children and adolescents. *J Paediatr Child Health* 2003; 39(6): 416-9.

Slater E, Beard AW. The schizophrenia-like psychoses of epilepsy, V: Discussion and conclusions. 1963. *Journal of Neuropsychiatry & Clinical Neurosciences* 1995; 7(3): 372-378.

Slettedal IO, Dahl HM, Sandvig I, Dalmau J, Stromme P. Young girl with psychosis, cognitive failure and seizures. *Tidsskr Nor Laegeforen* 2012; 132(18): 2073-6.

Vincent A, Bien CG, Irani SR, Waters P. Autoantibodies associated with diseases of the CNS: new developments and future challenges. *Lancet Neurol* 2011; 10(8): 759-72.

Wotton CJ, Goldacre MJ. Coexistence of schizophrenia and epilepsy: record-linkage studies. *Epilepsia* 2012; 53(4): e71-e74.

Youroukos S, Lazopoulou D, Michelakou D, Karagianni J. Acute psychosis associated with levetiracetam. *Epileptic Disord.* 2003; 5(2): 117-119.

Behavioural and psychiatric disorders associated with epilepsy syndromes

Frank Besag, Giuseppe Gobbi, Albert Aldenkamp,
Rochelle Caplan, David W. Dunn, Matti Sillanpää

Abstract

The categorisation of the childhood epilepsies into a number of different syndromes has allowed greater insight into the prognosis, not only with regard to seizure control but also in relation to cognitive and behavioural outcome. The role of genetics in determining both the syndrome and the behavioural outcome remains promising, although the promise is still largely unfulfilled. The behavioural/psychiatric outcome of a selection of the large number of childhood epilepsy syndromes is presented. The rate of autism in West syndrome, particularly in children who have tuberous sclerosis with temporal tubers, is high. In Dravet syndrome there is a loss of skills, with an associated increase in behavioural problems. The frequency of both subtle and overt seizures in the Lennox-Gastaut syndrome almost certainly accounts for the apparent poor motivation; however, a marked improvement in seizure control with treatment can also result in behavioural problems, probably as a result of the "release phenomenon". A number of cognitive problems can arise in the so-called "benign" syndrome of epilepsy with centrotemporal spikes (BECTS) and the rate of ADHD is high. Autistic features and ADHD have been described in the Landau-Kleffner syndrome and other syndromes associated with electrical status epilepticus of slow-wave sleep (ESES). Early effective treatment may reverse some of these features. There is clear evidence for a behavioural syndrome in relation to juvenile myoclonic epilepsy (JME), in which both clinical descriptions and functional neuroimaging indicate frontal lobe deficits.

Key words: West syndrome, Dravet syndrome, Lennox-Gastaut syndrome, Rolandic, Landau-Kleffner syndrome, juvenile myoclonic epilepsy

There has been an increasing recognition, over recent years, of the importance of the classification of childhood epilepsy into syndromes, not only to provide insight into the treatments that are most likely to be effective and the prognosis of the seizures but also with regard to the likely outcome in terms of cognition and behaviour. Because over 40 epilepsy syndromes and related conditions are listed in the proposed International League Against Epilepsy classification (Engel and International League Against Epilepsy, 2001), it is not possible to discuss the behavioural manifestations of each of these. Furthermore, the quality of behavioural information available is currently still limited. A few of the most frequently occurring and important syndromes will be discussed.

The importance of the behavioural implications of syndrome classification could be considered in two broad categories: first, the behavioural effects of epilepsy syndromes and second, the behavioural associations of childhood syndromes ("behavioural phenotypes") in which epilepsy occurs as a prominent feature. The second category includes a very large number of syndromes and will not be discussed here. However, in view of the extraordinary advances in genetics, particularly with the advent of array comparative genomic hybridization (array CGH), it is appropriate to draw attention to the growing number of genetic defects that are being recognised as being associated with epilepsy, intellectual disability and psychiatric problems. Galizia *et al.* (2012) examined adults with treatment-resistant epilepsy, most of whom had intellectual disability and at least some of whom had psychiatric disorders from childhood. The patients were drawn from two independent London hospitals. They identified copy number variants (CNVs) "judged to be of pathogenic significance" in 13.5% (7/52) and 20% (5/25) of the patients. These were on a variety of chromosomes including chromosomes 15 (four cases), 16 (three cases), 1, 9, 6 and 4. Bartnik *et al.* (2012) also found a large number of CNVs in their study of 102 patients with epilepsy, many of whom had developmental abnormalities. Battaglia and colleagues (2008; 2010) have drawn attention to the inv dup(15) or idic(15) syndrome, the clinical features of which include early central hypotonia, intellectual disability, autistic or autistic-like behaviour and epilepsy; seizures generally start between six months and nine years and a variety of seizure types can occur. Hesdorffer *et al.* (2012) examined familial clustering of epilepsy and behavioural disorders in 308 probands with childhood onset epilepsy. The DSM-oriented scales for affective disorder, anxiety disorder, conduct disorder and oppositional defiant disorder were significantly associated with a family history of unprovoked seizures. They concluded that their results supported the concept that behavioural disorders might be a manifestation of the underlying pathophysiology involved in the epilepsy.

With regard to the genetics of specific epilepsy syndromes, the situation remains that a single genetic defect can be associated with more than one syndrome and more than one genetic defect can be associated with a single syndrome. A discussion of the behavioural associations with specific epilepsy syndromes now follows. Descriptions of each of the syndromes will not be provided, because most of this information is available in a previous review (Besag, 2004).

■ Search strategy

The Medline/PubMed database was searched from inception until the end of March 2015 using the search terms: epilep$ and (child$ or pediat$ or adolescen$) and (behav$ or psychiat$ or psychol$) and ([name of syndrome]). Abstracts of likely relevance to the topic were examined to select papers for final detailed review. Reference lists of included papers were searched for any further relevant studies. The ILAE website section on epilepsy syndromes was examined for any further information.

West syndrome

The cognitive and behavioural outcome of West syndrome has been reviewed by Guzzetta (2006) and in other previous reviews of the behavioural outcome of epilepsy syndromes (Besag, 2004). Jambaque (1994) reviewed the neuropsychological outcome. Intellectual disability has typically been reported in around 70 to 80%. Riikonen and Amnell (1981) reported that 28% had psychiatric disorders with autism and hyperkinesis in equal numbers. The deterioration in cognition and behaviour appear to coincide with the onset of the severe EEG abnormality of hypsarrhythmia. Against this background, it might be expected that the cognitive and behavioural outcome would depend on prompt treatment. The study by O'Callaghan et al. (2011) on 77 infants showed clearly that the earlier the onset of the spasms and the longer the delay to treatment, the worse the outcome in terms of Vineland adaptive behaviour scales at 4 years of age.

There is a marked association between tuberous sclerosis and infantile spasms; the rate of autism in children who have both these conditions appears to be particularly high. For example, Hunt and Dennis (1987) stated that 58% of those who had both West syndrome and tuberous sclerosis remained autistic. When West syndrome occurs in babies with tuberous sclerosis the rate of seizure freedom with vigabatrin is very high. Jambaque et al. (2000) showed that when these babies were treated with vigabatrin both the mental age and the behaviour improved. Bolton et al. (2002) showed that autism is more likely to occur in children with tuberous sclerosis who had both infantile spasms and temporal lobe tubers, again suggesting that early treatment of the infantile spasms might improve not only cognition but also the psychiatric outcome. Similar conclusions were drawn from the study by Eisermann et al. (2003) for the treatment of infantile spasms in Down syndrome and by Bombardieri (2010) for babies who had tuberous sclerosis. There was a significant correlation between treatment lag, cessation of spasms and developmental quotient ($p = 0.003$) and with the score of autistic features ($p = 0.04$). For the group of patients who were treated within two months ($N = 8$), the response to treatment was more rapid ($p = 0.002$), the DQ was higher ($p = 0.004$) and the score of autistic features was lower ($p = 0.006$). All these studies give a clear indication that early treatment is more likely to be effective in terms of controlling the spasms and is also more likely to be associated with a better cognitive and psychiatric outcome.

Dravet syndrome (severe myoclonic epilepsy of infancy)

Brunklaus et al. (2011) carried out a study on quality of life and behavioural/psychiatric problems in 163 patients with Dravet syndrome. They screened for psychiatric/behavioural problems using the strengths and difficulties questionnaire (SDQ). The results were as follows: conduct problems 35%, hyperactivity/inattention 66% and peer relationship problems 76%. It should be noted, however, that the SDQ is not a particularly suitable instrument for children with more severe intellectual disability. Acha et al. (2014) found significant neurodevelopmental delay in patients with Dravet syndrome in both basic and higher-order cognitive performance. The impairment was greater in verbal abilities than in tasks that required processing visual material. Relative deficits in verbal abilities can influence both behaviour and the strategies used to manage behaviour. Nabbout et al. (2011) treated 15 patients with Dravet syndrome using the ketogenic diet; 66% had a decrease in seizure frequency of 75% or more. The authors said that not only was the seizure control improved but hyperactivity and behavioural disturbance also improved. This was a small study with promising results, suggesting that a larger trial would be worthwhile. Genton et al. (2011) carried out a long-term outcome study on 24 patients with Dravet syndrome. Five (21%) died. They commented that some patients "*had a major personality disorder, labelled autistic or psychotic*". Only three of the 24 patients lived independently. Because the seizures are often resistant to treatment, polytherapy tends to be used; Casse-Perrot et al. (2001) have commented that the polytherapy may contribute to the deterioration in cognition and behaviour. On the other hand, the deterioration in cognition and behaviour seems to coincide with the onset of EEG abnormalities, again raising the question of whether early effective treatment might lead to an improved outcome.

Lennox-Gastaut syndrome

Considering the severity of this syndrome, which involves frequent seizures of multiple types that are generally highly resistant to treatment, the data, both in terms of seizure outcome and behavioural disturbance remain extraordinarily sparse (Arzimanoglou et al., 2009; Cross and Neville, 2009; Hancock and Cross, 2009). Most of the studies have been on mixed groups of patients and have not used standardised behavioural measures. Mikati et al. (2009) assessed quality of life changes after vagus nerve stimulation in 16 patients with the Lennox-Gastaut syndrome, 11 of whom were children; the total group scored significantly higher in the social domain ($p = 0.039$). It is not surprising that they found that improvement in quality of life was significantly associated with seizure reduction ($p = 0.034$). Similar results were obtained in an earlier study by Majoie et al. (2001) on 16 children with "Lennox-like syndrome", who found that there were moderate improvements in mental functioning, behaviour and mood. Boyer and Deschatrette (1980) stated that a diagnosis of primary autism was made in nine children with the Lennox-Gastaut syndrome. Roger et al. (1987) carried out a large long-term study of 338 patients, who were followed into adulthood. They stated that 62.4% had an unfavourable outcome and that 20.4% had fairly rare partial seizures and neurological or psychiatric symptoms. Septien et al. (1992) found that two children with the Lennox-Gastaut syndrome had a frontal behavioural syndrome with hypokinesia, distractibility, aggressiveness and alexithymia; after they underwent an anterior two-thirds corpus callosotomy in the early teenage years they improved with regard to frontal-lobe syndrome features within two months of the surgery. Keiffer-Renaux et al. (2001) reported that behavioural problems were frequent in the first year of the seizure disorder; these problems were said to have included hypokinesia, with the inability to pursue an activity for more than a few minutes and autistic or psychotic features in some patients. It is highly likely that the hypokinesia described was a direct result of the frequent seizures that commonly occur in this syndrome. Some of the reports of behavioural disturbance when the seizure frequency is significantly decreased probably represent the "release phenomenon"; this situation can occur when someone who has been disabled by severe epilepsy for a long period becomes much more able as a result of successful seizure control but has not yet learned how to use their new-found ability in an acceptable way (Besag, 2001).

Benign childhood epilepsy with centrotemporal spikes (BECTS)/Rolandic epilepsy

Although this syndrome generally has a good outcome in terms of seizure control by the mid-teenage years, the previous impression that the outcome was also good in terms of behaviour and cognition was not accurate. There are now many papers demonstrating that a number of cognitive deficits and a significant rate of psychiatric disorder, especially ADHD, can occur in association with this syndrome (Heijbel and Bohman, 1975; D'Alessandro et al., 1990; Weglage et al., 1997; Staden et al., 1998; Croona et al., 1999; Massa et al., 2001; Giordani et al., 2006; Northcott et al., 2007; Taner et al., 2007; Lillywhite et al., 2009; Goldberg-Stern et al., 2010; Overvliet et al., 2011; Sarco et al., 2011; Genizi et al., 2012; Jurkeviciene et al., 2012; Raha et al., 2012; Filippini et al., 2013). It is also recognised that this syndrome lies on the spectrum with CSWS/Landau-Kleffner syndrome (Gobbi et al., 2006; Raha et al., 2012). Massa et al. (2001) have put forward the persuasive argument that the past statements that the syndrome was benign were based on retrospective studies that excluded children who did not have a benign outcome. They carried out a detailed prospective study on 35 children who fulfilled strict diagnostic criteria for BECTS. They were recruited immediately after the first seizure and were followed up for at least six months after the full normalisation of the EEG. In addition to carrying out a very detailed battery of psychometric tests, they classified educational performance impairments, behavioural disorders and social-familial problems into mild = 1, moderate = 2 or severe = 3. They then divided the 35 children into two groups: Group I with no relevant social-familial problems (score ≤ 2) and Group II who had developed serious difficulties impairing quality of life at home and at school (score ≥ 3). Group II had a poorer outcome on a wide variety of measurements, including educational performance, behavioural disorders, IQ during the course of the epilepsy, recovery IQ, auditory-verbal deficit, visual-spatial deficit and attention deficit. In particular, 10/25 (40%) in Group I had behavioural disorders (all mild, score = 1), whereas 10/10 (100%) in Group II had behavioural disorders (3 mild, 3 moderate and 4 severe). At onset, 4/25 (16%) of Group I had attention deficit compared with 8/10 (80%) of Group II. During the course of the epilepsy 10/25 (40%) of Group I had attention deficit (all mild) whereas 10/10 (100%) of Group II had attention deficit (2 mild, 4 moderate, 4 severe). In the recovery phase 5/25 (20%) in Group I had attention deficit (all mild) compared with 4/10 (40%) in Group II (2 mild, 2 severe).

Yung et al. (2000) examined the learning and behavioural problems of 78 children with centrotemporal spikes, 56 of whom had a history of clinical seizures compatible with BECTS and 22 of whom had centrotemporal spikes without clinical seizures. Eighteen of the 22 children who did not have clinical seizures were referred for psychiatric or behavioural problems and the other four were referred for suspected seizures that were not confirmed on video EEG monitoring. Three of the children had "atypical clinical features", including language disorder and regression. Eight out of the 78 (10%) had a borderline IQ (70-80), 7 (9%) had mild intellectual disability (IQ < 70). Twenty-four (31%) had behavioural problems, including inattention/distractibility, hyperactivity, aggression or oppositional behaviour. Thirteen (17%) had specific learning disability in reading, arithmetic or written expression, according to state of Georgia/South Carolina special education criteria. Forty-four of the 78 had neither behavioural nor learning difficulties. Three of the 78 had developmental or acquired aphasia; all three of these children had BECTS. In the group with BECTS, 12% had intellectual impairment, 14% had behavioural problems and 14% had a specific learning disability. It should be noted that the children without clinical seizures had a greater proportion of problems (36% intellectual impairment, 73% behavioural problems and 23% specific learning disability) but this is almost certainly because of the referral bias since those without obvious seizures were more likely to be referred because of behavioural/psychiatric problems. Referral bias is a limitation of this study but one of the strengths of the publication is the detailed information provided on a number of the individual cases.

Giordani et al. (2006) examined cognition and behaviour in 200 children with BECTS presenting for a trial of antiepileptic medication, implying that this was a selected group. The scores for all seizure groups were within the average range for intellectual and memory functioning. However, the simple partial seizure (focal seizure without impairment of awareness) group performed relatively worse on verbal learning. For those with complex partial (dyscognitive) seizures, parental report suggested greater psychosomatic and learning complaints.

Connelly et al. (2006) carried out a detailed neuropsychological common language and quality of life assessment in 30 children with BECTS. They used the Child Behaviour Checklist (CBCL), classifying behaviour into clinically abnormal, borderline clinical or normal, according to established methodology. The competence summary scores were: normal 72%, borderline 7% and abnormal 21% ($p < 0.0005$). The problem behaviour summary scores were: normal 67%, borderline 23% and abnormal 10% ($p = 0.016$) [The normative data for the Child Behaviour Checklist competence summary score are: borderline 3%, abnormal 2%. For problem behaviour, the normative data are borderline 8%, abnormal 10%]. Using the Child Health Questionnaire, the psychosocial summary score on 29 of the children revealed a mean of 41.41 (standard deviation 10.24, z-score -4.63, $p < 0.0005$) [For the Child Health Questionnaire the normative data mean is 50 with a standard deviation of 10].

Filippini et al. (2013) examined the longer-term effects of epileptiform discharges during non-rapid-eye-movement (NREM) sleep in 33 children with BECTS who were monitored for at least two years. They showed that the children were at higher risk for residual verbal difficulties and that the abnormal neuropsychological development was significantly correlated with a greater frequency of epileptiform discharges during NREM sleep. This might suggest that allowing such epileptiform discharges to continue long-term might also affect behaviour, although behavioural measures were not reported in this study.

Besseling et al. (2014) studied the structural and functional connectivity in BECTS. They found an impaired synergy between structural and functional development, especially in the youngest study subjects, suggesting delayed brain network maturation. The behavioural implications of these findings have yet to be determined.

The Landau-Kleffner syndrome

The acquired aphasia in the Landau-Kleffner syndrome occurs because of the development of verbal agnosia, apparently in association with electrical status epilepticus of slow-wave sleep or continuous spike-waves in slow-wave sleep (ESES/CSWS). It is not surprising that children who lose the ability to understand speech are liable to exhibit behavioural problems. A number of case reports and small series describe behavioural/psychiatric problems, including aggression, sleep disorders, hyperkinesia and autistic regression (Forster et al., 1983; White and Sreenivasan, 1987; Hirsch et al., 1990; Zivi et al., 1990;

Beaumanoir, 1992; Lopez-Ibor et al., 1997). Several papers have also discussed the relationship between autism, epileptiform discharges and the Landau-Kleffner syndrome (Nass et al., 1999; Tuchman, 2000; Deonna and Roulet, 2006; Besag, 2009). This subject has been reviewed by Deonna and Roulet-Perez in their book (2005). Nieuwenhuis and Nicolai (2006) reviewed the pathophysiological mechanisms of the cognitive and behavioural disturbances that can occur in this syndrome. Shinnar et al. (2001) prospectively identified 177 children with language regression, some of whom had the Landau-Kleffner syndrome, and stated that 88% met the criteria for autism or had autistic features. Overvliet et al. (2010) have reviewed the relationships between nocturnal seizures/epileptiform discharges and language impairment.

Several publications have emphasised the importance of early effective treatment. Medical treatments include steroids, sodium valproate, benzodiazepines, sulthiame and intravenous immunoglobulin. Surgical treatment with multiple subpial transection can be of great value when medical treatment has failed (*Behavioural effects of epilepsy surgery*, p. XX-XX). In the series published by Robinson et al. (2001), no child who had ESES for more than three years had a normal language outcome. This study, and a number of others, have indicated that the longer the ESES continues, the poorer the outcome in terms of language recovery and consequently the poorer of the outcome is likely to be in terms of behaviour. This implies that the longer the delay in providing early effective treatment, the more likely it will be that there will be long-term cognitive and behavioural problems. As discussed in previous reviews (Besag, 2004), this raises the question of when surgical intervention, in particular multiple subpial transection (Morrell et al., 1989), should be considered. Some children recover spontaneously, although there may be some residual language deficit, whereas others have permanent severe language deficits. If surgery is carried out too early, it may have been unnecessary but if it is carried out too late, the child may be left with serious problems that could have been avoided.

■ Other syndromes involving ESES or CSWS

The International League Against Epilepsy provides a description of a syndrome that involves CSWS or ESES but is not the Landau-Kleffner syndrome. An extract from the definition of "epilepsy with continuous spike-and-waves during slow-sleep (other than LKS)" follows. "*There is a constant and severe deterioration in neuropsychological functions associated with the disorder, and language capacity can be particularly affected. Patients may also show a profound decrease in intellectual level, poor memory, impaired temporospatial orientation, reduced attention span, hyperkinesis, aggressive behaviour, and even psychosis. Motor impairment, in the form of dyspraxia, dystonia, ataxia, or unilateral deficit, has been emphasised as one of the outstanding disturbances occurring in this syndrome. There is a strict association between the pattern of neuropsychological derangement and the location of the interictal focus...*"

The importance of this syndrome is the recognition that CSWS or ESES can present with a wide variety of deficits, not necessarily involving language – in contrast to the Landau-Kleffner syndrome. The similarity with the Landau-Kleffner syndrome is that CSWS or ESES occurs and may coincide with a marked deterioration in function that is, in at least some cases, reversible with antiepileptic medication or surgery (examples follow). The other characteristic that the two syndromes have in common is that obvious clinical seizures do not necessarily occur; although recognisable seizures are often part of the syndrome, the child may have a deterioration in function without having any current or past clinical seizures. The difference between the two syndromes, as already stated, is that language function is not necessarily involved in the CSWS syndrome.

Because ability may become acutely impaired in this syndrome, as for the Landau-Kleffner syndrome, it is not surprising that many of these children present with behavioural disturbance. Although several papers report behavioural disturbance that resolves with resolution of the CSWS, in most cases very few details of the behaviour itself are provided and, in general, standardised behavioural measures, during the acute phase of the CSWS and after this has resolved, are generally not available. Some of the reports that follow illustrate the variety of neurocognitive deficits that can occur in this syndrome.

Roulet-Perez et al. (1993) described an acquired epileptic frontal syndrome in four children with CSWS who had mental and behavioural regression. They commented that the pattern of behavioural and cognitive disturbance was similar to that found in some autistic-like disorders but they also drew attention to the similarity to the features of frontal lobe syndrome, more commonly described in adults. They made the important point that the deficits are potentially reversible and referred to the similarity to the Landau-Kleffner syndrome but with a different area of the brain being affected. Eriksson et al. (2003) described a striking case of visual agnosia accompanying occipito-temporal CSWS in an 8-year-old boy with sporadic seizures. There were no focal neurological signs. Visual acuity was intact. An MRI scan was normal. However, EEGs showed ESES/CSWS. Attention and executive functions were intact. There were no memory problems. He had normal global intelligence but major deficits in visual perception. Guzzetta et al. (2005) examined the cases of 32 patients with prenatal or perinatal thalamic injuries. Twenty-nine had "major sleep EEG activation". Twelve had CSWS. Behavioural problems were greater in patients with "true CSWS". Improvement in behaviour was in parallel with the disappearance of the CSWS. Aeby et al. (2005) assessed the effect of add-on levetiracetam on the EEG, behaviour and cognition of 12 patients with CSWS. In seven of the 12 (58%) the EEG was improved with the levetiracetam. Neuropsychological evaluation showed an improvement in three of the seven; the other four patients could not be tested because of the severity of the cognitive impairment. They commented that behaviour was improved in all seven patients. They also remarked that two patients improved in neuropsychological evaluation despite the lack of EEG improvement. Taner et al. (2007) carried out a detailed comparison study between 30 children with CSWS, 42 children with BECTS, 23 children with absence epilepsy and 40 healthy controls. There were high rates of ADHD (43.5-53.3%) and pervasive developmental disorder (43.5%-70%) in all the epilepsy groups, in sharp contrast to the control group. The most striking differences were in the high rate of intellectual disability in the CSWS group (33.3%) compared to the other two epilepsy groups: absence epilepsy (4.35%) and BECTS (11.9%). The rates of conduct disorder (27%) and anxiety disorders (30%) were also notably higher in the CSWS group than in the other groups but it should be noted that the overall numbers were small, implying that these differences should be viewed as being of doubtful significance. There were, however, statistically significant differences in all three WISC-R IQ measures (verbal IQ, performance IQ and full-scale IQ) between the CSWS group and both the absence group and the BECTS group. This raises the question of whether the higher rate of some of the psychiatric disorders in the CSWS group might have been accounted for, at least in part, by the lower cognitive ability of this group. Saltik et al. (2005) found that a number of clinical features indicated the development of ESES in a group of 16 children with idiopathic partial epilepsies. These features included an increase in seizure frequency, addition of new types of seizures, appearance of cognitive/behavioural changes or a progression in EEG abnormalities. Behavioural and psychiatric problems occurred in 81% (13/16); these included anxiety, depression, distractibility, hyperactivity, impulsivity and being easily frustrated. After remission of the ESES, three of the 13 patients had an excellent recovery, one was diagnosed as having the Landau-Kleffner syndrome, and nine patients performed better but did not achieve premorbid levels. Nikanorova et al. (2009) evaluated the ketogenic diet as treatment in five children (8-13 years of age) with CSWS refractory to conventional antiepileptic drugs and steroids. CSWS resolved in one patient. There was mild decrease in the spike-wave index in another patient. There was no response in the other three patients. The authors noted that, in two patients, there was an improvement in attention and behaviour. Kallay et al. (2009) demonstrated that an acquired frontal syndrome in association with CSWS was reversible by hemispherotomy at 5 years of age. Battaglia et al. (2009) similarly demonstrated that CSWS with refractory epilepsy from early injury to the thalamus resolved completely with functional hemispherectomy in two children, followed by progressive improvement in both cognition and behaviour. Seegmuller et al. (2012) carried out a long-term follow-up study of 10 adolescents and young adults who had had cognitive and behavioural regression with CSWS. The mean follow-up period was 15.6 years (range 8-23 years). None of the patients recovered fully but the marked behavioural disorders resolved in all but one of the 10. Three patients who had had a frontal syndrome during the active phase of CSWS had only mild residual executive and social cognition deficits. The outcome correlated with the duration of the CSWS, emphasising the recommendation that early effective treatment should be implemented.

The prominence of autistic features in association with CSWS has been emphasised by a number of workers (Tuchman, 2000; Deonna and Roulet, 2006). The classification of a specific acquired frontal syndrome with CSWS, as described in some of the reports presented earlier, has also been suggested (Roulet-Perez et al., 1993).

It is worth repeating that not all the children with CSWS have clinical seizures. The implication is that if cognition and behaviour deteriorate in a child, even if there is no history of seizures, unless another cause can be found, there is a strong argument for requesting overnight EEG monitoring.

Juvenile myoclonic epilepsy (Janz syndrome)

This has traditionally been considered to be a syndrome with a good outcome, both with regard to seizures (provided antiepileptic treatment is continued) and other aspects, despite the fact that the original publication by Janz and Christian (1957), over 50 years ago, confirmed more recently by Janz (2002), stated that many patients had attractive but unstable, suggestible and unreliable, rather immature personalities, often resulting in an inadequate social adjustment. Janz (2002) has pointed out that these features could be attributed to frontal lobe dysfunction and that neuroimaging studies appear to have confirmed this hypothesis. Risk-taking behaviour has been associated with microstructural alterations within frontal lobes of patients with juvenile myoclonic epilepsy (JME) (Wandschneider et al., 2013). Long-term follow up studies, for example the population-based study of Camfield and Camfield (2009), have indicated that some patients have seizures that are resistant to treatment and a number of studies have determined that a considerable proportion of those with JME have psychiatric/personality disorders (Janz and Christian, 1957; Trinka *et al.*, 2006; Moschetta *et al.*, 2011; de Araujo Filho *et al.*, 2013). By definition, this syndrome is not usually considered as presenting before around 12 years of age, although it appears that a proportion of children who have absence seizures subsequently develop JME. It would be of great interest to carry out a prospective study examining psychiatric and personality traits on a very large cohort of children with absence seizures to determine whether those who subsequently develop JME differ, with regard to their psychiatric profile, from those who do not. These data are currently sparse; most of the psychiatric data are on adults or mixed groups with relatively few teenagers. In a small sample of 19 children aged 8-18 years with new-onset JME, Lin *et al.* (2014) prospectively studied the maturational trajectories of brain and cognitive development in comparison with 57 healthy controls. At baseline, the cognitive abilities in the children with JME were similar to or worse than in controls; their cognitive abilities did not reach the level of healthy controls at two-year follow-up across most of the cognitive areas tested. MRI scans revealed significant abnormalities in cortical volume, thickness, and surface area in fronto-parieto-temporal regions. With regard to the personality traits, it might be reasonable to expect that the adult data would be of relevance to teenagers as well; the results from some studies have suggested that there might be grounds for this contention, *e.g.* Iqbal *et al.* (2009), whereas others do not, indicating that these traits might become more prominent with the duration of the epilepsy (see later). Psychiatric disorders such as psychosis, on the other hand, are likely to present in late adolescence or adulthood, often with no indication of pre-existing childhood or early teenage traits. For these reasons, the adult data on personality disorder will be presented but the adult data on other psychiatric disorders will, in general, not be discussed in this review. It should be noted that not all the papers have stated the age range of the population studied.

Perini *et al.* (1996) reported that the rate of psychiatric disorder in 18 patients with JME was 22%. Devinsky *et al.* (1997) carried out tests of frontal lobe functioning in 15 patients with JME who had a normal IQ; their performance was variable, with some patients showing marked impairment and others none. Concept formation-abstract reasoning and mental flexibility, cognitive speed and planning, and organisation were particularly affected. Gelisse *et al.* (2001) studied a mixed group of teenagers and adults (age range 15-70 years, mean 33 years) and found that 24 patients (15.5%) had persisting seizures despite adequate therapy and lifestyle. Psychiatric problems were strongly associated with seizure resistance: 58.3% in the resistant group compared with 19% in the non-resistant group ($p = 0.0026$). Trinka *et al.* (2006) also studied a mixed group of adults and teenagers (age range 15-63 years). They used the Structured Clinical Interviews for DSM-IV (SCID-I and SCID-II). 33% had one or more psychiatric disorder. Personality disorder was diagnosed in 23%. de Araujo Filho *et al.* (2007) compared the frequency of psychiatric disorders in 100 patients with JME compared with 100 healthy matched controls. They also used the DSM-IV SCID-I and SCID-II. Psychiatric disorders were diagnosed in 49 patients with JME. Anxiety disorder was diagnosed in 23 patients and mood disorder was diagnosed in 19 patients. Personality disorders were diagnosed in 17. The majority of these had cluster B personalities with the characteristics of impulsivity, humour reactivity, emotional instability and difficulty accepting social rules, factors that are remarkably similar to the original description by Janz and Christian (1957).

Plattner *et al.* (2007) used the Youth Self Report (YSR) and the Weinberger Adjustment Inventory (WAI) in 25 of 38 patients who agreed to participate and completed the assessments. The YSR revealed that JME patients had twice the amount of psychiatric symptoms compared to age-matched norms. Psychopathological symptoms increased with the duration of the JME. The WAI revealed decreased self-restraint; the longer the duration of the JME the less the self-control.

Iqbal et al. (2009) compared a group of eight sibling pairs, one of whom had JME and the other of whom did not, with 16 matched controls. The group of JME patients and their siblings differed significantly from controls on measures of phonemic and semantic verbal fluency and also scored significantly higher on the Dysexecutive Questionnaire, indicating that they were much more likely to have features associated with executive dysfunction. The authors interpreted these results as suggesting that both the patients and their siblings might have similar underlying dysfunction of cortical and subcortical structures responsible for these functions. It is interesting to compare these results with those of other studies, for example that of Plattner et al. (2007), that indicated that measures of frontal lobe dysfunction appeared to increase with the duration of the JME.

Pulsipher et al. (2009) compared 20 children with recent-onset JME with 51 healthy controls and 12 children with BECTS, using quantitative magnetic resonance imaging (MRI) and subtests from the Delis-Kaplan Executive Function System (D-KEFS) and the Behaviour Rating Inventory of Executive Function (BRIEF). They found that executive functions were impaired in the JME patients compared both to the controls and to the children with BECTS. The patients with JME had significantly smaller thalamic volumes and more frontal cerebrospinal fluid than controls and BECTS subjects.

de Araujo Filho et al. (2009b) carried out magnetic resonance spectroscopy studies comparing 16 JME patients who had cluster B personality disorders (see earlier) with 41 JME patients who had no psychiatric disorder and with 30 healthy controls. A significant reduction of the N-acetyl-aspartate/creatinine ratio was observed mainly in the left frontal lobe in the group of JME patients who had the personality disorder. The same group (de Araujo Filho et al., 2009a) carried out a volumetric MRI study in 16 JME patients with cluster B personality disorder compared with 38 patients without any psychiatric disorder and 30 matched healthy controls. Significant reductions were observed in the posterior region of the corpus callosum in the JME group with personality disorder relative to the other groups.

Guaranha et al. (2011) studied 65 consecutive JME patients, 45 of whom (61.5%) achieved good seizure control and 25 of whom (38.5%) became seizure free. They compared these with the remainder who had moderate or poor seizure control. Those with persistent seizures presented at a younger age at epilepsy onset (12.6 ± 3.33 years compared with 15.4 ± 5.47 years, $p = 0.015$) and had a higher prevalence of personality disorders (25% compared with 4%, $p = 0.029$) together with higher scores on the State-Trait Anxiety Inventory (45.9 ± 11.31 compared with 3.66 ± 11.43, $p = 0.011$).

Moschetta et al. (2011) examined personality traits in a mixed group of adults and teenagers, most of whom were adults (mean age 26.57 years, standard deviation 8.38) and 42 matched controls. They used the Temperament and Character Inventory (TCI). The JME patients had significantly higher scores on Novelty Seeking ($p = 0.001$) and Harm Avoidance ($p = 0.002$) and significantly lower scores on Self-Directedness ($p = 0.001$). They concluded that patients with JME had a higher expression of impulsive personality traits. The same group, Moschetta and Valente (2012), evaluated their 42 patients and a control group using the Digit Span tests (forwards and backwards), Stroop-Color Word Test, Trail Making Test, Wisconsin Card-Sorting Test, Matching Familiar Figures Test and Word

Fluency Test. The JME patients showed specific deficits in working memory, inhibitory control, concept formation, goal maintenance, mental flexibility and verbal fluency. Of the whole group of JME patients, 83% had moderate or severe executive dysfunction. Attention and executive impairment was correlated with a higher frequency of seizures and the presence of psychiatric disorders. Executive dysfunction correlated with a longer duration of epilepsy.

There is now a large body of evidence confirming the original observations of Janz and Christian (1957) that certain personality traits are much more common in patients with JME and that these reflect both structural and functional frontal lobe deficits. At what age these are present and to what extent other factors, such as duration and severity of the epilepsy, play a role remain subjects that require further investigation.

Conclusions

Although there is great variability within each of the childhood epilepsy syndromes, there is a growing body of evidence indicating that the identification of the epilepsy syndrome can be of prognostic value not only in terms of seizure control but also in providing an indication of the likely behavioural and cognitive outcome. This knowledge empowers clinicians and families, helping them to gain a greater understanding of the child as well as assisting in the planning of management and resources.

References

Acha, J., Perez, A., Davidson, D. J. & Carreiras, M. 2014. Cognitive characterization of children with Dravet syndrome: A neurodevelopmental perspective. *Child Neuropsychol*, 1-23.

Aeby, A., Poznanski, N., Verheulpen, D., Wetzburger, C. & Van, B. P. 2005. Levetiracetam efficacy in epileptic syndromes with continuous spikes and waves during slow sleep: experience in 12 cases. *Epilepsia*, 46, 1937-1942.

Arzimanoglou, A., French, J., Blume, W. T., Cross, J. H., Ernst, J. P., Feucht, M., Genton, P., Guerrini, R., Kluger, G., Pellock, J. M., Perucca, E. & Wheless, J. W. 2009. Lennox-Gastaut syndrome: a consensus approach on diagnosis, assessment, management, and trial methodology. *Lancet Neurology*, 8, 82-93.

Bartnik, M., Szczepanik, E. b., Derwi+äska, K., Wi+øniowieckaGÇÉKowalnik, B., Gambin, T., Sykulski, M., Ziemkiewicz, K., K-Ödzior, M., Gos, M. & HoffmanGÇÉZacharska, D. 2012. Application of array comparative genomic hybridization in 102 patients with epilepsy and additional neurodevelopmental disorders. *American Journal of Medical Genetics Part B: Neuropsychiatric Genetics*, 159, 760-771.

Battaglia, A. 2008. The inv dup (15) or idic (15) syndrome (Tetrasomy 15q). *Orphanet.J.Rare.Dis.*, 3, 30.

Battaglia, A., Parrini, B. & Tancredi, R. 2010. The behavioral phenotype of the idic(15) syndrome. *Am.J.Med.Genet.C.Semin.Med.Genet.*, 154C, 448-455.

Battaglia, D., Veggiotti, P., Lettori, D., Tamburrini, G., Tartaglione, T., Graziano, A., Veredice, C., Sacco, A., Chieffo, D., Pecoraro, A., Colosimo, C., Di, R. C., Dravet, C. & Guzzetta, F. 2009. Functional hemispherectomy in children with epilepsy and CSWS due to unilateral early brain injury including thalamus: sudden recovery of CSWS. *Epilepsy Res.*, 87, 290-298.

Beaumanoir, A. 1992. The Landau-Kleffner Syndrome. In: ROGER, J., BUREAU, M., DRAVET, C., DREIFUSS, F. E., PERRET, A. & WOLF, P. (eds.) *Epileptic syndromes in infancy, childhood and adolescence.* Second ed. London: John Libbey & Company Limited.

Besag, F. M. C. 2001. Behavioural effects of the new anticonvulsants. *Drug Safety*, 24, 513-536.

Besag, F. M. C. 2004. Behavioral aspects of pediatric epilepsy syndromes. *Epilepsy & Behavior*, 5, Suppl-13.

Besag, F. M. C. 2009. The relationship between epilepsy and autism: a continuing debate. *Acta Paediatrica*, 98, 618-620.

Besseling, R. M., Jansen, J. F., Overvliet, G. M., van der Kruijs, S. J., Ebus, S. C., de Louw, A. J., Hofman, P. A., Aldenkamp, A. P. & Backes, W. H. 2014. Delayed convergence between brain network structure and function in rolandic epilepsy. *Front Hum Neurosci*, 8, 704.

Bolton, P. F., Park, R. J., Higgins, J. N., Griffiths, P. D. & Pickles, A. 2002. Neuro-epileptic determinants of autism spectrum disorders in tuberous sclerosis complex. *Brain*, 125, 1247-1255.

Bombardieri, R., Pinci, M., Moavero, R., Cerminara, C. & Curatolo, P. 2010. Early control of seizures improves long-term outcome in children with tuberous sclerosis complex. *European Journal of Paediatric Neurology*, 14, 146-149.

Boyer, J. P. & Deschatrette, A. 1980. Convulsive autism or Lennox-Gastaut syndrome? Apropos of 9 cases of primary autism associated with Lennox-Gastaut syndrome [French]. *Neuropsychiatrie de l Enfance et de l Adolescence*, 28, 93-100.

Brunklaus, A., Dorris, L. & Zuberi, S. M. 2011. Comorbidities and predictors of health-related quality of life in Dravet syndrome. *Epilepsia*, 52, 1476-1482.

Camfield, C. S. & Camfield, P. R. 2009. Juvenile myoclonic epilepsy 25 years after seizure onset: a population-based study. *Neurology*, 73, 1041-1045.

Casse-Perrot, C., Wolf, M. & Dravet, C. 2001. Neuropsychological aspects of severe myoclonic epilepsy in infancy. In: JAMBAQUE, I., LASSONDE, M. & DULAC, O. (eds.) *Neuropsychology of Childhood Epilepsy.* New York: Kluwer Academic/Plenum Publishers.

Connolly, A. M., Northcott, E., Cairns, D. R., McIntyre, J., Christie, J., Berroya, A., Lawson, J. A., Bleasel, A. F. & Bye, A. M. 2006. Quality of life of children with benign rolandic epilepsy. *Pediatric Neurology*, 35, 240-245.

Croona, C., Kihlgren, M., Lundberg, S., Eeg-Olofsson, O. & Eeg-Olofsson, K. E. 1999. Neuropsychological findings in children with benign childhood epilepsy with centrotemporal spikes. *Developmental Medicine & Child Neurology*, 41, 813-818.

Cross, J. H. & Neville, B. G. 2009. The surgical treatment of Landau-Kleffner syndrome. *Epilepsia*, 50 Suppl 7, 63-67.

D'Alessandro, P., Piccirilli, M., Tiacci, C., Ibba, A., Maiotti, M., Sciarma, T. & Testa, A. 1990. Neuropsychological features of benign partial epilepsy in children. *Ital.J.Neurol.Sci.*, 11, 265-269.

de Araujo Filho, G. M., de Araujo, T. B., Sato, J. R., Silva, I., Lin, K., Junior, H. C., Yacubian, E. M. & Jackowski, A. P. 2013. Personality traits in juvenile myoclonic epilepsy: evidence of cortical abnormalities from a surface morphometry study. *Epilepsy Behav.*, 27, 385-392.

de Araujo Filho, G. M., Jackowski, A. P., Lin, K., Guaranha, M. S., Guilhoto, L. M., da Silva, H. H., Caboclo, L. O., Junior, H. C., Bressan, R. A. & Yacubian, E. M. 2009a. Personality traits related to juvenile myoclonic epilepsy: MRI reveals prefrontal abnormalities through a voxel-based morphometry study. *Epilepsy Behav.*, 15, 202-207.

de Araujo Filho, G. M., Lin, K., Lin, J., Peruchi, M. M., Caboclo, L. O., Guaranha, M. S., Guilhoto, L. M., Carrete, H., Jr. & Yacubian, E. M. 2009b. Are personality traits of juvenile myoclonic epilepsy related to frontal lobe dysfunctions? A proton MRS study. *Epilepsia*, 50, 1201-1209.

de Araujo Filho, G. M., Pascalicchio, T. F., Sousa, P. S., Lin, K., Ferreira Guilhoto, L. M. & Yacubian, E. M. 2007. Psychiatric disorders in juvenile myoclonic epilepsy: a controlled study of 100 patients. *Epilepsy Behav.*, 10, 437-441.

Deonna, T. & Roulet-Perez, E. 2005. *Cognitive and behavioural disorders of epileptic origin in children*, Cambridge, Mac Keith Press/Cambridge University Press.

Deonna, T. & Roulet, E. 2006. Autistic spectrum disorder: evaluating a possible contributing or causal role of epilepsy. *Epilepsia*, 47 Suppl 2, 79-82.

Devinsky, O., Gershengorn, J., Brown, E., Perrine, K., Vazquez, B. & Luciano, D. 1997. Frontal functions in juvenile myoclonic epilepsy. *Neuropsychiatry, Neuropsychology, & Behavioral Neurology*, 10, 243-246.

Eisermann, M. M., DeLaRaillere, A., Dellatolas, G., Tozzi, E., Nabbout, R., Dulac, O. & Chiron, C. 2003. Infantile spasms in Down syndrome: effects of delayed anticonvulsive treatment. *Epilepsy Research*, 55, 21-27.

Engel, J., Jr. & International League Against Epilepsy 2001. A proposed diagnostic scheme for people with epileptic seizures and with epilepsy: report of the ILAE Task Force on Classification and Terminology. *Epilepsia*, 42, 796-803.

Eriksson, K., Kylliainen, A., Hirvonen, K., Nieminen, P. & Koivikko, M. 2003. Visual agnosia in a child with non-lesional occipito-temporal CSWS. *Brain Dev.*, 25, 262-267.

Filippini, M., Boni, A., Giannotta, M. & Gobbi, G. 2013. Neuropsychological development in children belonging to BECTS spectrum: long-term effect of epileptiform activity. *Epilepsy Behav.*, 28, 504-511.

Forster, C., Braun, H. & Weidner, G. 1983. Aphasia with epilepsy: a new syndrome? [German]. *Monatsschrift Kinderheilkunde*, 131, 788-792.

Galizia, E. C., Srikantha, M., Palmer, R., Waters, J. J., Lench, N., Ogilvie, C. M., Kasperavi-ìi+$^1/_2$t-ù, D., Nashef, L. & Sisodiya, S. M. 2012. Array comparative genomic hybridization: Results from an adult population with drug-resistant epilepsy and co-morbidities. *European Journal of Medical Genetics*, 55, 342-348.

Gelisse, P., Genton, P., Samuelian, J. C., Thomas, P. & Bureau, M. 2001. Psychiatric disorders in juvenile myoclonic epilepsy [French]. *Revue Neurologique*, 157, 297-302.

Genizi, J., Shamay-Tsoory, S. G., Shahar, E., Yaniv, S. & Aharon-Perez, J. 2012. Impaired social behavior in children with benign childhood epilepsy with centrotemporal spikes. *Journal of Child Neurology*, 27, 156-161.

Genton, P., Velizarova, R. & Dravet, C. 2011. Dravet syndrome: the long-term outcome. *Epilepsia*, 52, Suppl-9.

Giordani, B., Caveney, A. F., Laughrin, D., Huffman, J. L., Berent, S., Sharma, U., Giles, J. M. & Garofalo, E. A. 2006. Cognition and behavior in children with benign epilepsy with centrotemporal spikes (BECTS). *Epilepsy Research*, 70, 89-94.

Gobbi, G., Boni, A. & Filippini, M. 2006. The spectrum of idiopathic Rolandic epilepsy syndromes and idiopathic occipital epilepsies: from the benign to the disabling. *Epilepsia*, 47, Suppl-6.

Goldberg-Stern, H., Gonen, O. M., Sadeh, M., Kivity, S., Shuper, A. & Inbar, D. 2010. Neuropsychological aspects of benign childhood epilepsy with centrotemporal spikes. *Seizure*, 19, 12-16.

Guaranha, M. S., Filho, G. M., Lin, K., Guilhoto, L. M., Caboclo, L. O. & Yacubian, E. M. 2011. Prognosis of juvenile myoclonic epilepsy is related to endophenotypes. *Seizure*, 20, 42-48.

Guzzetta, F. 2006. West syndrome. *Epilepsia*, In press.

Guzzetta, F., Battaglia, D., Veredice, C., Donvito, V., Pane, M., Lettori, D., Chiricozzi, F., Chieffo, D., Tartaglione, T. & Dravet, C. 2005. Early thalamic injury associated with epilepsy and continuous spike-wave during slow sleep. *Epilepsia*, 46, 889-900.

Hancock, E. C. & Cross, H. H. 2009. Treatment of Lennox-Gastaut syndrome. *Cochrane Database of Systematic Reviews*, CD003277.

Heijbel, J. & Bohman, M. 1975. Benign epilepsy of children with centrotemporal EEG foci: intelligence, behavior, and school adjustment. *Epilepsia*, 16, 679-687.

Hesdorffer, D. C., Caplan, R. & Berg, A. T. 2012. Familial clustering of epilepsy and behavioral disorders: evidence for a shared genetic basis. *Epilepsia*, 53, 301-307.

Hirsch, E., Marescaux, C., Maquet, P., Metz-Lutz, M. N., Kiesmann, M., Salmon, E., Franck, G. & Kurtz, D. 1990. Landau-Kleffner syndrome: a clinical and EEG study of five cases. *Epilepsia*, 31, 756-767.

Hunt, A. & Dennis, J. 1987. Psychiatric disorder among children with tuberous sclerosis. *Developmental Medicine & Child Neurology*, 29, 190-198.

Iqbal, N., Caswell, H. L., Hare, D. J., Pilkington, O., Mercer, S. & Duncan, S. 2009. Neuropsychological profiles of patients with juvenile myoclonic epilepsy and their siblings: a preliminary controlled experimental video-EEG case series. *Epilepsy Behav.*, 14, 516-521.

Jambaque, I. 1994. Neuropsychological Aspects. *In:* DULAC, O., CHUGANI, H. T. & DALLA BERNADINA, B. (eds.) *Infantile Spasms and West Syndrome*. London: W. B. Saunders Company Ltd.

Jambaque, I., Chiron, C., Dumas, C., Mumford, J. & Dulac, O. 2000. Mental and behavioural outcome of infantile epilepsy treated by vigabatrin in tuberous sclerosis patients. *Epilepsy Research*, 38, 151-160.

Janz, D. 2002. The psychiatry of idiopathic generalized epilepsy. *In:* TRIMBLE, M. & SCHMITZ, B. (eds.) *The Neuropsychiatry of Epilepsy*. Cambridge: Cambridge University Press.

Janz, D. & Christian, W. 1957. Impulsiv-Petit mal. *Dtch Z Nervenheilk*, 176, 346-386.

Jurkeviciene, G., Endziniene, M., Laukiene, I., Saferis, V., Rastenyte, D., Plioplys, S. & Vaiciene-Magistris, N. 2012. Association of language dysfunction and age of onset of benign epilepsy with centrotemporal spikes in children. *European Journal of Paediatric Neurology*, 16, 653-661.

Kallay, C., Mayor-Dubois, C., Maeder-Ingvar, M., Seeck, M., Debatisse, D., Deonna, T. & Roulet-Perez, E. 2009. Reversible acquired epileptic frontal syndrome and CSWS suppression in a child with congenital hemiparesis treated by hemispherotomy. *Eur.J.Paediatr.Neurol.*, 13, 430-438.

Kieffer-Renaux, V., Kaminska, A. & Dulac, O. 2001. Cognitive deterioration in Lennox-Gastaut and Doose epilepsy. *In:* JAMBAQUE, I., LASSONDE, M. & DULAC, O. (eds.) *Neuropsychology of Childhood Epilepsy*. New York: Kluwer Academic/Plenum Publishers.

Lillywhite, L. M., Saling, M. M., Harvey, A. S., Abbott, D. F., Archer, J. S., Vears, D. F., Scheffer, I. E. & Jackson, G. D. 2009. Neuropsychological and functional MRI studies provide converging evidence of anterior language dysfunction in BECTS. *Epilepsia*, 50, 2276-2284.

Lin, J. J., Dabbs, K., Riley, J. D., Jones, J. E., Jackson, D. C., Hsu, D. A., Stafstrom, C. E., Seidenberg, M. & Hermann, B. P. 2014. Neurodevelopment in new-onset juvenile myoclonic epilepsy over the first 2 years. *Ann Neurol*, 76, 660-8.

Lopez-Ibor, M. I., Lopez-Ibor, J. J. & Hernandez, H. M. 1997. Landau-Kleffner syndrome (acquired aphasia with epilepsy). Etiopathology and response to treatment with anticonvulsants [Spanish]. *Actas Luso-Espanolas de Neurologia, Psiquiatria y Ciencias Afines*, 25, 410-416.

Majoie, H. J., Berfelo, M. W., Aldenkamp, A. P., Evers, S. M., Kessels, A. G. & Renier, W. O. 2001. Vagus nerve stimulation in children with therapy-resistant epilepsy diagnosed as Lennox-Gastaut syndrome: clinical results, neuropsychological effects, and cost-effectiveness. *Journal of Clinical Neurophysiology*, 18, 419-428.

Massa, R., Saint-Martin, A., Carcangiu, R., Rudolf, G., Seegmuller, C., Kleitz, C., Metz-Lutz, M. N., Hirsch, E. & Marescaux, C. 2001. EEG criteria predictive of complicated evolution in idiopathic rolandic epilepsy. *Neurology*, 57, 1071-1079.

Mikati, M. A., Ataya, N. F., El-Ferezli, J. C., Baghdadi, T. S., Turkmani, A. H., Comair, Y. G., Kansagra, S. & Najjar, M. W. 2009. Quality of life after vagal nerve stimulator insertion. *Epileptic Disorders*, 11, 67-74.

Morrell, F., Whisler, W. W. & Bleck, T. P. 1989. Multiple subpial transection: a new approach to the surgical treatment of focal epilepsy. *Journal of Neurosurgery*, 70, 231-239.

Moschetta, S., Fiore, L. A., Fuentes, D., Gois, J. & Valente, K. D. 2011. Personality traits in patients with juvenile myoclonic epilepsy. *Epilepsy Behav.*, 21, 473-477.

Moschetta, S. P. & Valente, K. D. 2012. Juvenile myoclonic epilepsy: the impact of clinical variables and psychiatric disorders on executive profile assessed with a comprehensive neuropsychological battery. *Epilepsy Behav.*, 25, 682-686.

Nabbout, R., Copioli, C., Chipaux, M., Chemaly, N., Desguerre, I., Dulac, O. & Chiron, C. 2011. Ketogenic diet also benefits Dravet syndrome patients receiving stiripentol: a prospective pilot study. *Epilepsia*, 52, e54-e57.

Nass, R., Gross, A., Wisoff, J. & Devinsky, O. 1999. Outcome of multiple subpial transections for autistic epileptiform regression. *Pediatric Neurology*, 21, 464-470.

Nieuwenhuis, L. & Nicolai, J. 2006. The pathophysiological mechanisms of cognitive and behavioral disturbances in children with Landau-Kleffner syndrome or epilepsy with continuous spike-and-waves during slow-wave sleep. [Review] [76 refs]. *Seizure*, 15, 249-258.

Nikanorova, M., Miranda, M. J., Atkins, M. & Sahlholdt, L. 2009. Ketogenic diet in the treatment of refractory continuous spikes and waves during slow sleep. *Epilepsia*, 50, 1127-1131.

Northcott, E., Connolly, A. M., Berroya, A., McIntyre, J., Christie, J., Taylor, A., Bleasel, A. F., Lawson, J. A. & Bye, A. M. 2007. Memory and phonological awareness in children with Benign Rolandic Epilepsy compared to a matched control group. *Epilepsy Research*, 75, 57-62.

O'Callaghan, F. J., Lux, A. L., Darke, K., Edwards, S. W., Hancock, E., Johnson, A. L., Kennedy, C. R., Newton, R. W., Verity, C. M. & Osborne, J. P. 2011. The effect of lead time to treatment and of age of onset on developmental outcome at 4 years in infantile spasms: evidence from the United Kingdom Infantile Spasms Study. *Epilepsia*, 52, 1359-1364.

Overvliet, G. M., Aldenkamp, A. P., Klinkenberg, S., Nicolai, J., Vles, J. S., Besseling, R. M., Backes, W., Jansen, J. F., Hofman, P. A. & Hendriksen, J. 2011. Correlation between language impairment and problems in motor development in children with rolandic epilepsy. *Epilepsy & Behavior*, 22, 527-531.

Overvliet, G. M., Besseling, R. M., Vles, J. S., Hofman, P. A., Backes, W. H., van Hall, M. H., Klinkenberg, S., Hendriksen, J. & Aldenkamp, A. P. 2010. Nocturnal epileptiform EEG discharges, nocturnal epileptic seizures, and language impairments in children: review of the literature. *Epilepsy & Behavior*, 19, 550-558.

Perini, G. I., Tosin, C., Carraro, C., Bernasconi, G., Canevini, M. P., Canger, R., Pellegrini, A. & Testa, G. 1996. Interictal mood and personality disorders in temporal lobe epilepsy and juvenile myoclonic epilepsy. *Journal of Neurology, Neurosurgery & Psychiatry*, 61, 601-605.

Plattner, B., Pahs, G., Kindler, J., Williams, R. P., Hall, R. E., Mayer, H., Steiner, H. & Feucht, M. 2007. Juvenile myoclonic epilepsy: a benign disorder? Personality traits and psychiatric symptoms. *Epilepsy Behav.*, 10, 560-564.

Pulsipher, D. T., Seidenberg, M., Guidotti, L., Tuchscherer, V. N., Morton, J., Sheth, R. D. & Hermann, B. 2009. Thalamofrontal circuitry and executive dysfunction in recent-onset juvenile myoclonic epilepsy. *Epilepsia*, 50, 1210-1219.

Raha, S., Shah, U. & Udani, V. 2012. Neurocognitive and neurobehavioral disabilities in Epilepsy with Electrical Status Epilepticus in slow sleep (ESES) and related syndromes. *Epilepsy Behav.*, 25, 381-385.

Riikonen, R. & Amnell, G. 1981. Psychiatric disorders in children with earlier infantile spasms. *Developmental Medicine & Child Neurology*, 23, 747-760.

Robinson, R. O., Baird, G., Robinson, G. & Simonoff, E. 2001. Landau-Kleffner syndrome: course and correlates with outcome. *Developmental Medicine & Child Neurology*, 43, 243-247.

Roger, J., Remy, C., Bureau, M., Oller-Daurella, L., Beaumanoir, A., Favel, P. & Dravet, C. 1987. Lennox-Gastaut syndrome in the adult [French]. *Revue Neurologique*, 143, 401-405.

Roulet-Perez, E., Davidoff, V., Despland, P. A. & Deonna, T. 1993. Mental and behavioural deterioration of children with epilepsy and CSWS: acquired epileptic frontal syndrome. *Developmental Medicine & Child Neurology*, 35, 661-674.

Saltik, S., Uluduz, D., Cokar, O., Demirbilek, V. & Dervent, A. 2005. A clinical and EEG study on idiopathic partial epilepsies with evolution into ESES spectrum disorders. *Epilepsia*, 46, 524-533.

Sarco, D. P., Boyer, K., Lundy-Krigbaum, S. M., Takeoka, M., Jensen, F., Gregas, M. & Waber, D. P. 2011. Benign rolandic epileptiform discharges are associated with mood and behavior problems. *Epilepsy & Behavior*, 22, 298-303.

Seegmuller, C., Deonna, T., Dubois, C. M., Valenti-Hirsch, M. P., Hirsch, E., Metz-Lutz, M. N., de Saint, M. A. & Roulet-Perez, E. 2012. Long-term outcome after cognitive and behavioral regression in nonlesional epilepsy with continuous spike-waves during slow-wave sleep. *Epilepsia*, 53, 1067-1076.

Septien, L., Giroud, M., Sautreaux, J. L., Brenot, M., Marin, A., Dumas, R. & Nivelon, J. L. 1992. Effects of callosotomy in the treatment of intractable epilepsies in children on psychiatric disorders [French]. *Encephale*, 18, 199-202.

Shinnar, S., Rapin, I., Arnold, S., Tuchman, R. F., Shulman, L., Ballaban-Gil, K., Maw, M., Deuel, R. K. & Volkmar, F. R. 2001. Language regression in childhood. *Pediatric Neurology*, 24, 183-189.

Staden, U., Isaacs, E., Boyd, S. G., Brandl, U. & Neville, B. G. 1998. Language dysfunction in children with Rolandic epilepsy. *Neuropediatrics*, 29, 242-248.

Taner, Y., Erdogan-Bakar, E., Turanli, G. & Topcu, M. 2007. Psychiatric evaluation of children with CSWS (continuous spikes and waves during slow sleep) and BRE (benign childhood epilepsy with centrotemporal spikes/rolandic epilepsy) compared to children with absence epilepsy and healthy controls. *Turkish Journal of Pediatrics*, 49, 397-403.

Trinka, E., Kienpointner, G., Unterberger, I., Luef, G., Bauer, G., Doering, L. B. & Doering, S. 2006. Psychiatric comorbidity in juvenile myoclonic epilepsy. *Epilepsia*, 47, 2086-2091.

Tuchman, R. 2000. Treatment of seizure disorders and EEG abnormalities in children with autism spectrum disorders. *Journal of Autism & Developmental Disorders*, 30, 485-489.

Wandschneider, B., Centeno, M., Vollmar, C., Stretton, J., O'Muircheartaigh, J., Thompson, P. J., Kumari, V., Symms, M., Barker, G. J., Duncan, J. S., Richardson, M. P. & Koepp, M. J. 2013. Risk-taking behavior in juvenile myoclonic epilepsy. *Epilepsia*, 54, 2158-65.

Weglage, J., Demsky, A., Pietsch, M. & Kurlemann, G. 1997. Neuropsychological, intellectual, and behavioral findings in patients with centrotemporal spikes with and without seizures. *Developmental Medicine & Child Neurology*, 39, 646-651.

White, H. & Sreenivasan, U. 1987. Epilepsy-aphasia syndrome in children: an unusual presentation to psychiatry. *Canadian Journal of Psychiatry – Revue Canadienne de Psychiatrie*, 32, 599-601.

Yung, A. W., Park, Y. D., Cohen, M. J. & Garrison, T. N. 2000. Cognitive and behavioral problems in children with centrotemporal spikes. *Pediatric Neurology*, 23, 391-395.

Zivi, A., Broussaud, G., Daymas, S., Hazard, J. & Sicard, C. 1990. Epilepsy-acquired aphasia syndrome with psychosis. Report of a case [French]. *Annales de Pediatrie*, 37, 391-394.

Subtle behavioural and cognitive manifestations of epilepsy

Frank Besag, Giuseppe Gobbi, Albert Aldenkamp, Rochelle Caplan, David W. Dunn, Matti Sillanpää

Abstract

A subtle behavioural or cognitive manifestation of epilepsy can be defined in two ways. First, epileptiform discharges not presenting as obvious seizures may nevertheless affect cognition and/or behaviour. Second, the actual seizures may be obvious but the way they affect cognition or behaviour may not be. There is a growing body of evidence indicating that the epileptiform discharges in benign epilepsy with centrotemporal spikes can affect behaviour and cognition. The focal discharges in other forms of epilepsy can also be associated with behavioural change. The Landau-Kleffner syndrome, the CSWS syndrome, transitory cognitive impairment and transient epileptic amnesia provide further examples of cognitive and behavioural manifestations resulting from subtle manifestations of the epilepsy. Prompt, effective antiepileptic treatment with medication or surgery can improve behaviour and cognition in at least some cases.

Key words: Rolandic, centrotemporal, absence, transitory, ESES, CSWS

Although some authors have, over many years, drawn attention to the importance of subtle manifestations of epilepsy in affecting the behaviour and cognition of children with epilepsy (Marston, 1992; Marston et al., 1993; Aldenkamp, 1997; Deonna and Roulet-Perez, 2005; Binnie and Besag, 2011), it is perhaps the growing number of papers reporting such effects in the syndrome of benign epilepsy with centrotemporal spikes (BECTS) (see later) that has provided compelling evidence. This raises the controversial issue of whether children with epileptiform discharges in the EEG but who are not necessarily having obvious seizures should be treated with antiepileptic medication (Besag, 1995). However, there are other situations, apart from BECTS, in which subtle manifestations of epilepsy can affect behaviour and cognition. This topic has been reviewed elsewhere (Besag, 2011). The current paper will draw on previous reviews, as well as discussing some of the more recent data.

Search strategy

In addition to papers already known to the authors, the Medline/PubMed database was searched from inception until the end of March 2015 using the search terms: epilep$ and (child$ or adolescen$) and (subtle or ESES or CSWS or TCI or transitory cognitive impairment). Abstracts of likely relevance to the topic were examined to select papers for final detailed review. Reference lists of included papers were searched for any further relevant studies.

Definitions

A subtle behavioural or cognitive effect of epilepsy has been defined as an effect that is not immediately obviously attributable to an epileptic seizure (Besag, 2011). This does not necessarily imply that the epileptic activity itself is "subtle". For example, some children have very frequent nocturnal seizures; although the seizures might be obvious (if someone is awake to observe them), the fact that the child is tired, irritable or functions poorly the following day because of this nocturnal epileptic activity might not be correctly attributed to the seizures. In other cases the epileptic activity itself is subtle. The classical example is the child with absence seizures, who might not be recognised as having epileptic seizures at all, although these might not only affect behaviour and function but can also have safety implications (Wirrell et al., 1996). Examples of subtle behavioural manifestations of epilepsy include not only absence seizures but also transitory cognitive impairment, frequent localised epileptiform discharges, electrical status epilepticus of slow wave sleep (ESES) or continuous spike-wave discharges in slow-wave sleep (CSWS), transient epileptic amnesia and postictal effects. Some of these examples will be discussed in more detail. These are all examples of what has been termed "state-dependent impairment", a concept that has been defined elsewhere (Besag, 2011). In summary, state-dependent cognitive or behavioural impairment is potentially treatable and reversible, in contrast to permanent impairment, which is not. The most recent system of epilepsy classification (Berg and Millichap, 2013) has drawn attention to the concept of "epileptic encephalopathy", in which the epileptiform discharges themselves can affect cognition and behaviour. Debate about the terminology continues; some might prefer to reserve the term "encephalopathy" for conditions in which a clearer structural or metabolic brain pathology can be identified.

Frequent absence seizures

In the past it has been suggested that children with absence seizures have no behavioural or cognitive problems. The publication by Caplan et al. (2008) on 69 children with absence seizures reported a high rate of both cognitive and behavioural disturbance. These data have been confirmed by Masur et al. (2013), Thio (2013) and Bernson-Leung and Mazumdar (2014). Furthermore, EEG monitoring has shown that some children have not only hundreds of spike-wave episodes per day but, in some cases, thousands of such episodes daily (Besag, 2011). These can have a major effect on their ability to interact with the world around them, with both behavioural and cognitive consequences.

Frequent localised discharges

Frequent left temporal discharges have been associated with aggressive behaviour. Surgical removal of the focus can result in marked behavioural improvement. Serafetinides (1965) reported on 100 consecutive temporal lobectomy patients at the Maudsley Hospital, the majority of whom had childhood-onset epilepsy and underwent the surgery under 19 years of age. They compared aggressive and non-aggressive patients; there was a predominance of left temporal epileptiform foci in the aggressive group. In several cases the surgery cured not only the epilepsy but also the aggression. However, no convincing replication of these results could be found and one recent study failed to confirm this finding (Andresen et al., 2014).

Frequent frontal discharges can be associated with a major deterioration in behaviour; in the experience of at least one of the authors, surgical removal of an active left frontal epileptiform focus can result in a major improvement in behaviour, although further evidence for this is required. Some support is provided by the recent favourable outcome following frontal lobe resections in children reported by Andresen et al. (2014). A related, but apparently clinically distinct situation has been described by Fohlen et al. (2004), who described "behavioural epileptic seizures" in eight children with frontal lobe epilepsy. They carried out prolonged, invasive video-EEG monitoring in this group of children. The "behavioural epileptic seizures" manifested as a variety of clinical phenomena, including mood change, sudden agitation, unexpected quietness and subtle change of awareness on awakening. The children had a number of other seizure manifestations, some of which were more obvious and some which were not, including clonic facial/eyelid movements, head and eye deviation, staring, drop attacks, facial erythema, smiling, laughing and apnoea.

The best documented situation of surgical treatment of frequent localised epileptiform discharges is that of surgical treatment of children or teenagers with an abnormal cerebral hemisphere as the source of such discharges. Either anatomical or functional hemispherectomy have been reported as resulting in major behavioural improvements, in well-established reviews (Goodman, 1986; Lindsay et al., 1987; Pulsifer et al., 2004).

Van Bogaert et al. (2012) reported that functional neuroimaging evidence suggests that interictal epileptiform discharges may impact cognition, either through transient effects on brain processing mechanisms or through more long-lasting effects, leading to prolonged inhibition of brain areas distant from, but connected with the epileptic focus (i.e. a remote inhibition effect). Sustained interictal epileptiform discharges may also impair sleep-related learning consolidation processes.

Transitory cognitive impairment

This phenomenon has been described and reported in detail, notably by Binnie and colleagues (Aarts et al., 1984; Binnie and Marston, 1992). An epileptiform discharge that does not appear to be manifesting as an obvious seizure can cause transitory impairment of cognitive function. It has been shown (in left-hemisphere-dominant individuals) that left-sided discharges can impair language function and right-sided discharges can impair visuo-spatial function (Aarts et al., 1984). It has also been shown that transitory cognitive impairment can affect psychosocial function (Marston et al., 1993). In an extensive review of the literature, Aldenkamp and Arends (2004) concluded that the concept of transitory cognitive impairment (which they term "transient cognitive impairment") was still valid, but a refinement of methodology had shown that a large proportion of presumed transitory cognitive impairment could be attributed to subtle seizures, while interictal epileptic activity accounts for a much smaller part of the cognitive effects than previously thought. This opens the debate on what constitutes an epileptic seizure. If the latter is defined as any clinical manifestation of an epileptiform discharge then transitory cognitive impairment is another example of subtle seizure activity. Gonzalez-Garrido et al. (2000) examined transitory cognitive impairment in 58 children with epilepsy, aged 8 to 12 years compared with 20 healthy children. Paroxysmal discharges in the EEGs were found in 87.9% and 5% of the two groups, respectively. Transitory cognitive impairment was detected in 36.2% of the children with epilepsy. Fonseca et al. (2007) assessed transitory cognitive impairment in 33 children with benign childhood epilepsy with centrotemporal spikes. Only two of the children made a significantly greater proportion of errors during the rolandic spikes. They concluded that transitory cognitive impairment occured in only a limited number of their cases and did not impair school performance. More recently, Nair et al. (2014) evaluated the EEGs of 60 consecutive children with focal or interictal spike-and-wave discharges using power spectral analysis to determine if there were any changes in power spectra that continued after the interictal abnormalities. They concluded that effects of interictal activity on EEG rhythms appear to be transient and confined to the duration of the interictal discharge; interictal EEG discharges seem temporarily to alter neural activity during the duration of the spike-and-wave discharge but there was no evidence that alterations of spectral power continued immediately beyond the duration of the discharge.

■ Transient epileptic amnesia and accelerated long-term forgetting

The initial reports of transient epileptic amnesia were in adults (Butler et al., 2009). It presents as recurrent transient episodes of memory loss; it can be associated with accelerated long-term forgetting (ALF) and autobiographical memory loss. Gascoigne et al. (2012) demonstrated that children with idiopathic generalized epilepsy (IGE) may present with ALF, which is related to epilepsy severity. They suggested that their findings might support the notion that the epilepsy or the seizures themselves might disrupt long-term memory consolidation. In another study, Gascoigne et al. (2014) compared 23 children with temporal lobe epilepsy (TLE) and 58 healthy controls of similar age, sex distribution and socioeconomic status. They reported evidence of ALF in children with TLE, which could not be explained by poor performance on standard memory tests. Additionally, these authors suggested that the developmental trajectory of long-term memory in children with TLE is similar to that of short-term memory and that deficits emerge gradually, implying that older children are more likely to present with long-term memory deficits.

■ Electrical status epilepticus of slow wave sleep (ESES) or continuous spike-waves of slow-wave sleep (CSWS)

The best-known example of major behavioural and cognitive changes occurring in association with ESES is the Landau-Kleffner syndrome of acquired epileptic aphasia (Landau and Kleffner, 1957). This syndrome usually presents after language acquisition but before 6 years of age. The child loses the ability to recognise speech (verbal auditory agnosia), which may be followed by a more generalised auditory agnosia with the inability to recognise environmental sounds as well. Expressive language can be profoundly affected, probably because the child cannot understand his or her own speech. The waking EEG typically has frequent multifocal epileptiform discharges, usually in the temporal areas. The overnight EEG may show electrical status epilepticus of slow-wave sleep (ESES), in which at least 85% of slow-wave sleep is replaced by spike-wave discharges. Approximately 30% of children with the Landau-Kleffner syndrome do not have a history of obvious seizures but do have the EEG abnormalities. The seizures usually resolve by the early to mid-teenage years but the language recovery is very variable; some individuals are left with profound language impairment (Fandino et al., 2011; Caraballo et al., 2014). It is not surprising that a number of behavioural disturbances have been described in this syndrome, including autistic features and features of attention deficit hyperactivity disorder.

The International League Against Epilepsy recognises a syndrome of CSWS which can present with major impairment in abilities other than language (Subtle behavioural and cognitive manifestations of epilepsy in children, p. xx-xx). The suggestion in older publications was that the cognitive and behavioural impairments in children with the Landau-Kleffner syndrome (and, by implication, children with other impairments associated with ESES/CSWS) are not amenable to antiepileptic treatment. The evidence over recent years has shown that this is not the case. Medical treatment with steroids, sodium valproate, levetiracetam sulthiame, benzodiazepines and immunoglobulin can be effective in at least some cases (Kramer et al., 2009). The surgical technique of multiple subpial transection, developed by Frank Morrell (1989), can result in dramatic improvement in speech. However, if treatment is delayed, the outcome is unlikely to be very favourable, as shown by Robinson et al. (2001).

The role of slow-wave sleep in normal cortical plasticity during critical developmental periods has recently been reviewed by Issa (2014). He discussed how disruption of slow-wave sleep by electrographic seizures could affect cortical maps and the development, organization and functional connectivity of the thalamic structures. Bolsterli Heinzle et al. (2014), in a retrospective study, calculated the slope of slow waves (0.5-2 Hz) in the first hour and last hour of sleep of 14 patients with CSWS. The authors reported that there was no overnight change of the slope of slow waves in the "focus", while in "nonfocal" regions the slope decreased significantly. This difference in the overnight course resulted in a steeper slope in the "focus" compared to "nonfocal" electrodes during the last hour of sleep. Spike-wave density was correlated with the impairment of the overnight slope decrease: the higher the spike-wave density, the more hampered the slope decrease. Since the overnight decrease of the slope was shown to be closely related to the recovery function of sleep, and such recovery is necessary for optimal cognitive performance during wakefulness, the authors suggested that the impairment of this process by spike-waves is a potential mechanism leading to neuropsychological deficits in CSWS.

Conclusion

The effect of subtle manifestations can be profound. Recognition of these effects of epilepsy, followed by early, effective treatment might avoid many of the associated cognitive and behavioural problems.

References

Aarts, J. H., Binnie, C. D., Smit, A. M. & Wilkins, A. J. 1984. Selective cognitive impairment during focal and generalized epileptiform EEG activity. *Brain*, 107, 293-308.

Aldenkamp, A. P. 1997. Effect of seizures and epileptiform discharges on cognitive function. *Epilepsia*, 38, S52-S55.

Aldenkamp, A. P. & Arends, J. 2004. Effects of epileptiform EEG discharges on cognitive function: is the concept of "transient cognitive impairment" still valid? *Epilepsy Behav*, 5 Suppl 1, S25-34.

Andresen, E. N., Ramirez, M. J., Kim, K. H., Dorfman, A. B., Haut, J. S., Klaas, P. A., Jehi, L. E., Shea, K., Bingaman, W. E. & Busch, R. M. 2014. Effects of surgical side and site on mood and behavior outcome in children with pharmacoresistant epilepsy. *Front Neurol*, 5, 18.

Berg, A. T. & Millichap, J. J. 2013. The 2010 revised classification of seizures and epilepsy. *Continuum (Minneap.Minn.)*, 19, 571-597.

Bernson-Leung, M. E. & Mazumdar, M. 2014. Journal club: pretreatment EEG in childhood absence epilepsy. *Neurology*, 82, e158-60.

Besag, F. M. C. 1995. The therapeutic dilemma: treating subtle seizures or indulging in electroencephalogram cosmetics? *Seminars in Pediatric Neurology*, 2, 261-268.

Besag, F. M. C. 2011. Subtle cognitive and behavioral effects of epilepsy. *In*: TRIMBLE, M. & SCHMITZ, B. (eds.) *The Neuropsychiatry of Epilepsy*. 2nd ed. Cambridge, UK: Cambridge University Press.

Binnie, C. D. & Marston, D. 1992. Cognitive correlates of interictal discharges. *Epilepsia*, 33, S11-S17.

Bolsterli Heinzle, B. K., Fattinger, S., Kurth, S., Lebourgeois, M. K., Ringli, M., Bast, T., Critelli, H., Schmitt, B. & Huber, R. 2014. Spike wave location and density disturb sleep slow waves in patients with CSWS (continuous spike waves during sleep). *Epilepsia*, 55, 584-91.

Butler, C. R., Bhaduri, A., Acosta-Cabronero, J., Nestor, P. J., Kapur, N., Graham, K. S., Hodges, J. R. & Zeman, A. Z. 2009. Transient epileptic amnesia: regional brain atrophy and its relationship to memory deficits. *Brain*, 132, 2-68.

Caplan, R., Siddarth, P., Stahl, L., Lanphier, E., Vona, P., Gurbani, S., Koh, S., Sankar, R. & Shields, W. D. 2008. Childhood absence epilepsy: behavioral, cognitive, and linguistic comorbidities. *Epilepsia*, 49, 1838-1846.

Caraballo, R. H., Cejas, N., Chamorro, N., Kaltenmeier, M. C., Fortini, S. & Soprano, A. M. 2014. Landau-Kleffner syndrome: a study of 29 patients. *Seizure*, 23, 98-104.

Deonna, T. & Roulet-Perez, E. 2005. *Cognitive and behavioural disorders of epileptic origin in children*, Cambridge, Mac Keith Press/Cambridge University Press.

Fandino, M., Connolly, M., Usher, L., Palm, S. & Kozak, F. K. 2011. Landau-Kleffner syndrome: a rare auditory processing disorder series of cases and review of the literature. *International Journal of Pediatric Otorhinolaryngology*, 75, 33-38.

Fohlen, M., Bulteau, C., Jalin, C., Jambaque, I. & Delalande, O. 2004. Behavioural epileptic seizures: a clinical and intracranial EEG study in 8 children with frontal lobe epilepsy. *Neuropediatrics*, 35, 336-345.

Fonseca, L. C., Tedrus, G. M. & Pacheco, E. M. 2007. Epileptiform EEG discharges in benign childhood epilepsy with centrotemporal spikes: reactivity and transitory cognitive impairment. *Epilepsy Behav*, 11, 65-70.

Gascoigne, M. B., Barton, B., Webster, R., Gill, D., Antony, J. & Lah, S. S. 2012. Accelerated long-term forgetting in children with idiopathic generalized epilepsy. *Epilepsia*, 53, 2135-40.

Gascoigne, M. B., Smith, M. L., Barton, B., Webster, R., Gill, D. & Lah, S. 2014. Accelerated long-term forgetting in children with temporal lobe epilepsy. *Neuropsychologia*, 59, 93-102.

Gonzalez-Garrido, A. A., Oropeza de Alba, J. L., Gomez-Velazquez, F. R., Fernandez Harmony, T., Soto Mancilla, J. L., Ceja Moreno, H., Perez Rulfo, D., Gonzalez Cornejo, S., Riestra Castneda, R., Aguirre Portillo, L. E., Gomez Limon, E. & Ruiz Sandoval, J. L. 2000. Transitory cognitive impairment in epileptic children during a CPT task. *Clin Electroencephalogr*, 31, 175-80.

Goodman, R. 1986. Hemispherectomy and its alternatives in the treatment of intractable epilepsy in patients with infantile hemiplegia. *Developmental Medicine & Child Neurology*, 28, 251-258.

Issa, N. P. 2014. Neurobiology of continuous spike-wave in slow-wave sleep and Landau-Kleffner syndromes. *Pediatr Neurol*, 51, 287-96.

Kramer, U., Sagi, L., Goldberg-Stern, H., Zelnik, N., Nissenkorn, A. & Ben-Zeev, B. 2009. Clinical spectrum and medical treatment of children with electrical status epilepticus in sleep (ESES). *Epilepsia*, 50, 1517-1524.

Landau, W. M. & Kleffner, F. R. 1957. Syndrome of acquired aphasia with convulsive disorder in children. *Neurology (Minneap.)*, 7, 523-530.

Lindsay, J., Ounsted, C. & Richards, P. 1987. Hemispherectomy for childhood epilepsy: a 36-year study. *Developmental Medicine & Child Neurology*, 29, 592-600.

Marston, D., Besag, F. M. C., Binnie, C. D. & Fowler, M. 1993. Effects of transitory cognitive impairment on psychosocial functioning of children with epilepsy: a therapeutic trial. *Developmental Medicine & Child Neurology*, 35, 574-581.

Masur, D., Shinnar, S., Cnaan, A., Shinnar, R. C., Clark, P., Wang, J., Weiss, E. F., Hirtz, D. G., Glauser, T. A. & Childhood Absence Epilepsy Study, G. 2013. Pretreatment cognitive deficits and treatment effects on attention in childhood absence epilepsy. *Neurology*, 81, 1572-80.

Morrell, F., Whisler, W. W. & Bleck, T. P. 1989. Multiple subpial transection: a new approach to the surgical treatment of focal epilepsy. *Journal of Neurosurgery*, 70, 231-239.

Nair, S., Morse, R. P., Mott, S. H., Burroughs, S. A. & Holmes, G. L. 2014. Transitory effect of spike and spike-and-wave discharges on EEG power in children. *Brain Dev*, 36, 505-9.

Pulsifer, M. B., Brandt, J., Salorio, C. F., Vining, E. P., Carson, B. S. & Freeman, J. M. 2004. The cognitive outcome of hemispherectomy in 71 children. *Epilepsia*, 45, 243-254.

Robinson, R. O., Baird, G., Robinson, G. & Simonoff, E. 2001. Landau-Kleffner syndrome: course and correlates with outcome. *Developmental Medicine & Child Neurology*, 43, 243-247.

Serafetinides, E. A. 1965. Aggressiveness in temporal lobe epileptics and its relation to cerebral dysfunction and environmental factors. *Epilepsia*, 6, 33-42.

Thio, L. L. 2013. Childhood absence epilepsy: poor attention is more than seizures. Neurology, 81, e138-9.

Van Bogaert, P., Urbain, C., Galer, S., Ligot, N., Peigneux, P. & De Tiege, X. 2012. Impact of focal interictal epileptiform discharges on behaviour and cognition in children. *Neurophysiol Clin*, 42, 53-8.

Wirrell, E. C., Camfield, P. R., Camfield, C. S., Dooley, J. M., Gordon & KE. 1996. Accidental injury is a serious risk in children with typical absence epilepsy. Archives of Neurology, 53, 929-932.

Adverse cognitive and behavioural effects of antiepileptic drugs in children

Albert Aldenkamp, Frank Besag, Giuseppe Gobbi,
Rochelle Caplan, David W. Dunn, Matti Sillanpää

Abstract

The literature was evaluated for cognitive and more general behavioural effects. We distinguished the older antiepileptic drugs (AEDs), from the newer and newest AEDs. The striking finding was the lack of information on children. From the available evidence it would appear that there may be negative cognitive effects with phenobarbital, phenytoin, topiramate and zonisamide, and adverse behavioural effects with phenobarbital, valproate, gabapentin, topiramate, levetiracetam and zonisamide. There is inconclusive data on ethosuximide, clobazam, vigabatrin, felbamate, pregabalin, stiripentol, rufinamide, lacosamide and retigabine. The following drugs appear to be neutral with regard to cognitive effects: valproate, carbamazepine, gabapentin and oxcarbazepine. Carbamazepine appears to be neutral with regard to behavioural effects. Positive cognitive effects have been reported with lamotrigine and levetiracetam. Positive behavioural effects have been reported with lamotrigine. Recommendations are provided.

Key words: antiepileptic drug, cognition, attention, memory

■ Search strategy

PubMed was searched for all articles before up to January 2015 using the Medical Subject Heading (MeSH) terms "Antiepileptic drugs", "Epilepsy", "Behaviour", "Cognition". Also, in combination with "Cognition and Behaviour", all individual AEDs were entered. Limits were set at: "All child 0-16 years" and "English". Case reports were subsequently removed.

Older AEDs

Phenobarbital (PB)

PB has been used for the treatment of epilepsy since the discovery of its antiepileptic effect by Hauptman in 1912 (Kumbier and Haack, 2002). The main antiepileptic mechanism of action is the increase of the duration (not the frequency) of GABA-activated chloride ion channel opening, hence potentiating GABA-mediated inhibitory neurotransmission. PB can also activate the $GABA_A$ receptor in the absence of GABA, which is sometimes considered to be a mechanism leading to its sedative properties (Kwan and Brodie, 2004).

One study reported no difference in global cognitive function, as measured with the Wechsler Preschool and Primary Scale of Intelligence (WPPSI), between PB and placebo (Wolf et al., 1981). However, baseline testing before the start of treatment was not performed; the children were tested before the drug was discontinued and again approximately three months later. IQ, measured using the Bayley Scales, was significantly lower in the PB group in toddler-aged children randomly assigned to receive long-term (two years) PB or placebo for febrile seizures (Farwell et al., 1990). Six months later, after drug discontinuation, normalisation was established. Three to five years later, when these children had entered school and were retested, there were no differences in IQ between those who had been treated with PB and the placebo group (Sulzbacher et al., 1999). However, the PB group scored lower than the placebo group on the reading achievement from the Wide Range Achievement Test (WRAT-R).

Cognitive and behavioural effects of PB in toddlers were assessed in a randomized, placebo-controlled study of those who had had a febrile seizure (Camfield et al., 1979). After eight to 12 months of therapy there were no differences in IQ, as measured by the Bayley scales, between PB and placebo. However, there were some effects of PB on memory and on comprehension. Greater serum levels and length of treatment had a negative impact on performance. Parents reported behavioural changes in 43% of toddlers taking PB compared with 20% taking placebo. Parents complained about increased fussiness and a disturbance of sleep (waking up in the middle of the night). Hyperactivity was not seen in this study. However, Wolf and Forsythe (1978) found that 42% of the children treated with PB developed a behaviour disorder, usually hyperactivity.

In comparison with valproic acid, lower performance was seen on measurements of cognitive function and behaviour (Vining et al., 1987; Calandre et al., 1990). After six months of treatment, children performed less well on tests of neuropsychological function, in particular with respect to memory, while receiving PB (Vining et al., 1987). After 9-12 months of treatment, the increase found in IQ scores for controls and VPA was not found for PB (Calandre et al., 1990). Parental assessment of behaviour of 21 children indicated impaired behaviour for PB; children with PB were measurably more hyperactive (Vining et al., 1987).

Compared to children treated with CBZ, children with newly-diagnosed partial onset seizures treated with PB did not differ on measures of cognitive function or behaviour at six-month and 12 month follow-up (Mitchell and Chavez, 1987). The behavioural effect of PB was also compared with placebo in children under 2 years of age. Changes in behaviour were assessed with a standard questionnaire completed by each mother three and nine weeks after starting the drug (Bacon et al., 1981). There were no differences in behavioural outcomes between PB, phenytoin and placebo. However, after drug discontinuation, children who had been taking PB exhibited more behavioural problems, in particular uncooperative and demanding behaviour, compared with children who discontinued PHT or placebo.

In a study in rural India, no differences in behavioural problems were also reported by Pal et al. (1998) in comparison to PHT. Behavioural adverse effects were assessed with the Conners parent rating scale for children 6 years of age and above and with the preschool behavioural screening questionnaire for younger children. The frequency of behavioural problems was 30% in both treatment groups.

In conclusion, the most convincing studies revealed negative effects on both cognition and behaviour. A broad range of cognitive functions was affected, including higher-order functions such as memory. Some studies even suggested that intelligence was impaired by PB. The behavioural problems reported ranged from hyperactivity to withdrawal or sedation.

Phenytoin (PHT)

PHT has been used as an antiepileptic drug since it was first developed in 1938 by Merritt and Putnam. For 20 years PHT was (together with PB) the universal treatment for epilepsy. PHT has excellent antiepileptic properties and is used as a relatively broad-spectrum AED. The main antiepileptic mechanism of action is use-dependent (voltage-dependent and frequency-dependent) sodium channel blocking. PHT binds to the fast inactivated state of the channel, reducing high-frequency neuronal firing. PHT has a stronger effect on the sodium channel than CBZ, delaying recovery more than CBZ. PHT may also have mild effects on the excitatory glutamate system and on the inhibitory GABA system.

Aldenkamp et al. (1993) used a drug-withdrawal design and showed more impairment, specifically more slowing of central information processing, for PHT compared to CBZ in children with Rolandic epilepsy. Forsythe et al. (1991) randomly assigned 64 children to carbamazepine, phenytoin or valproate. Cognition was assessed before commencing the drug and during treatment. They reported that carbamazepine in moderate dosage affected memory but this effect was not found with either phenytoin or valproate.

Bacon et al. (1981) compared the behavioural effects of PHT to placebo in children under 2 years of age. Changes in behaviour were assessed using a standard questionnaire completed by each mother, three and nine weeks after starting the drug. At nine weeks, fewer children taking PHT were reported as being shy or as having fears about things than those taking placebo.

In conclusion, in contrast to reports in adults, the cognitive and behavioural effects of PHT seem to be limited. This opens the possibility that the reported effects of PHT, such as slowing of central information processing speed (Aldenkamp et al., 1993) are chronic effects that only occur after long treatment periods.

Ethosuximide (ESX)

ESX was introduced in 1960 and has mainly been used for the treatment of generalized absence seizures. ESX modifies the properties of voltage-dependent calcium channels, reducing the T-type currents, thereby preventing synchronized firing. The reduction is most prominent at negative membrane potentials and less prominent at more positive membrane potentials. Most of the effect is assumed to take place in thalamocortical relay neurons (Broicher et al., 2007).

Glauser et al. (2010; 2013) compared ESX to VPA and LTG. They concluded that ESX is the optimal choice for initial monotherapy in childhood absence epilepsy. ESX was associated with fewer adverse attentional effects, as measured with the Conners Continuous Performance Test, compared to VPA, both after short-term (16-20 weeks) and long-term (one year) treatment.

In conclusion, there is very little information about the positive or negative cognitive or behavioural effects of ESX, despite clinical experience for over half a century.

Carbamazepine (CBZ)

CBZ was first synthesized in the early 1950s and introduced as an antiepileptic drug by Bonduelle in 1964 (Shorvon, 2009) in Europe. CBZ is used for treating complex partial (dyscognitive) seizures, with or without secondary generalization. Approval by the FDA for use in the United States followed much later (1978) because of concerns about serious haematological toxicity, namely aplastic anaemia (Donaldson and Graham, 1965). The main antiepileptic mechanism of action is similar to that of PHT with a less "slowing" effect in the recovery state than obtained for PHT. The mechanism of action is also voltage-dependent and frequency-dependent.

Neurocognitive performance was evaluated in seven children with symptomatic localisation-related epilepsy who were seizure-free for at least two years. They were tested prior to and at least 12 months after discontinuation of CBZ (Riva and Devoti, 1999). Results indicated that CBZ did not affect intellectual, memory or attentional functions, or more complex frontal functions. Nevertheless, after therapy withdrawal, scores on frontal function tests improved. The authors suggested that these functions might have been better without CBZ therapy.

In a study by Forsythe et al. (1991) 64 children with newly-diagnosed tonic-clonic or partial seizures (aged 5 to 14 years) were randomly assigned to treatment with CBZ, PHT or VPA. A control group was also included. The children were assessed with cognitive tests before starting medication and at one, six and 12 months after starting treatment. CBZ adversely affected memory, but VPA and PHT did not.

However, Trimble and Cull (1988) reported better reaction times and scores on various cognitive tests in children taking CBZ compared with those taking VPA. Stores et al. (1992) evaluated the cognitive and behavioural effects of VPA and CBZ in 63 children with newly-diagnosed epilepsy compared to controls. They were tested before starting treatment and one month, six months and one year after starting treatment, on standardised tests of intelligence, school attainments, attention, memory and visuomotor function, together with parent and teacher questionnaire information about various aspects of behaviour. CBZ and VPA were equivalent, in being associated with no reduction in intelligence or school attainments over the first 12 months of treatment. Attentional differences were more consistently seen throughout the repeated assessments, with lower sustained attention scores characterising the CBZ group. In addition, poorer performance than controls was seen on the pegboard measure of visuomotor coordination, early in the treatment with CBZ. Behaviour questionnaires showed that at three and six months into treatment the CBZ group, surprisingly, had lower inattention scores than controls (described by the authors as being an anomalous result) but at 12 months of treatment no differences were found.

When barbiturates (PB) were withdrawn in 45 children because of chronic behavioural difficulties and replaced by CBZ, general alertness and attentiveness were improved four to six months later (Schain et al., 1977).

Berg et al. (1993) randomly assigned 64 new cases of childhood epilepsy to CBZ, PHT or VPA. Behavioural measures were assessed before medication and after one and six months of treatment. Those treated with CBZ and VPA had minor behavioural difficulties after one month of treatment, but these did not persist at six months.

Eun et al. (2012) compared the behavioural effects of CBZ to LTG as monotherapy for paediatric epilepsy. Sixty-seven previously untreated children with partial-onset seizures were treated with CBZ or LTG and followed for 24 weeks. Externalizing behaviour problems improved in patients taking CBZ but there were no differences between the two groups. The parent report on the Conners scale showed an improvement for carbamazepine compared to lamotrigine. Based on this study, CBZ had a more favourable behavioural profile than LTG.

In conclusion, there is much evidence that treatment with CBZ is not complicated by serious adverse cognitive or behavioural effects in children.

Sodium valproate (VPA)

VPA, a fatty acid, appears to have multiple mechanisms of action (Loscher, 2002). Several studies have demonstrated an effect on sodium channels that is different from PHT or CBZ. An effect on T-type calcium channels has also been demonstrated. Recent studies have, however, shown that a predominant effect concerns the interaction with the GABAergic neurotransmitter system. VPA may augment GABA release and block the re-uptake of GABA into glial cells. VPA elevates brain GABA levels and potentiates GABA responses, possibly by enhancing GABA synthesis and inhibiting degradation. Theoretically, such mechanisms of action could cause cognitive adverse effects. VPA is one of the most effective drugs against generalized absence seizures.

In comparison to PB, differences were seen on measurements of cognitive function and behaviour in favour of VPA (Vining et al., 1987; Calandre et al., 1990). Children receiving PB performed worse than those receiving VPA on cognitive measurements, particularly intelligence and memory. Furthermore, parental assessment of behaviour indicated worse behaviour for PB; more hyperactivity was reported for PB than for VPA. In comparison to PHT, no differences were found (Forsythe et al., 1991). In comparison to CBZ, children treated with VPA had slower reaction times (Trimble and Cull, 1988). Poorer performance than controls was seen on the more complex digit symbol task during the middle phase of the 12-month period of treatment with VPA and lower focal attention scores on cognitive tests (Stores et al., 1992). VPA negatively affected attention, as measured with the Conners Continuous Performance Test, to a greater degree than did either LTG or ESX (Glauser et al., 2010). Berg et al. (1993) found that CBZ and VPA were associated with minor behavioural difficulties after one month of treatment, but these problems were not present at six months of treatment.

In conclusion, there are few studies on the behavioural and cognitive effects of VPA. There is insufficient information to confirm the clinical impression that VPA is sometimes associated with behavioural problems.

Clobazam (CLB)

CLB was reported to have antiepileptic activity by Gastaut (1978). It is a 1,5 benzodiazepine which was initially developed as an anxiolytic drug.

In a randomized, double-blind prospective study, the cognitive and behavioural effects of CLB were studied in comparison to standard monotherapy of childhood epilepsy. Children with newly-diagnosed epilepsy were assigned randomly to receive CLB, CBZ or PHT. Neuropsychological assessments were compared at six weeks and 12 months after commencing the study medication. There were no differences between the CLB and standard monotherapy groups on measures of intelligence, memory, psychomotor speed, attention or impulsivity in the initial assessment carried out when the dosage of medication had been stabilized (after six weeks), or on the neuropsychological measures at the one-year follow-up assessment. A checklist of systemic and behavioural adverse effects was completed by the attending paediatric neurologist, based on spontaneous and elicited parental reports and physical examination at study entry and at each follow-up visit at six weeks and 12 months. Behavioural adverse effects were characterized as externalizing (e.g. restless, aggressive) or internalizing (e.g. depressed, withdrawn) in nature. There were no differences in the frequency of internalizing or externalizing behavioural adverse effects between the CLB and standard monotherapy groups. The authors concluded that the cognitive and behavioural effects of CLB were comparable to those of standard monotherapy (Bawden et al., 1999).

In children treated with CLB for refractory epilepsy, 11% developed a severe behaviour disorder which was characterized by aggressive agitation, self-injurious behaviour, insomnia and incessant motor activity. Most of the affected children were developmentally disabled (Sheth et al., 1994).

Jan and Shabat (2000) in a later study of CLB for refractory epilepsy in 31 children (21M 10F, 2 months to 15 years of age, mean 4.6 years), reported adverse effects including excessive sedation, vomiting, irritability, behavioural change and ataxia in seven (22.5%).

In conclusion, the few controlled data for CLB do not indicate that it is associated with serious cognitive effects, although behavioural effects have been reported.

■ Newer AEDs

Vigabatrin (VGB)

VGB is an irreversible inhibitor of the GABA-transaminase. It is one of the most effective agents for treating infantile spasms and refractory complex partial (dyscognitive) seizures (Marson et al., 1997). Its clinical use is limited because of the frequent occurrence of peripheral visual field defects (Eke et al., 1997; Kalviainen et al., 1999).

A review of the literature on VGB reported an incidence of severe abnormal behaviour in controlled trials in around 6% in children (Ferrie et al., 1996).

Thirteen children underwent psychometric and behavioural evaluation before VGB initiation and at a mean of three years on VGB treatment to evaluate the long-term cognitive outcome of children whose refractory spasms definitely disappeared when VGB was given as an add-on drug (Jambaque et al., 2000). The cessation of spasms with VGB was associated with significant improvement of cognition and behaviour in these children with tuberous sclerosis.

In the United Kingdom Infantile Spasms Study (UKISS) neurodevelopment was assessed with the Vineland adaptive behaviour scales (VABS) in children randomly assigned to hormone treatment or VGB. At 12-14 months of age the mean VABS scores did not differ between the two treatments. In infants with no identified underlying aetiology, the mean VABS score was higher in those allocated to hormone treatment than in those allocated to VGB (Lux et al., 2005). This difference persisted at 4 years of age: in those infants with no identified aetiology, the VABS remained higher for those allocated to hormonal treatment than for those allocated to VGB (Darke et al., 2010). Increasing waiting time to treatment was associated with decreasing developmental score at four years in all infants with infantile spasms after adjustment for the effects of aetiology and treatment allocation (O'callaghan et al., 2011). This research group suggested that early identification with prompt diagnosis and treatment of infants with infantile spasms may help to prevent subsequent developmental delay and improve developmental outcome.

In conclusion, the interpretation of the behavioural data for VGB is complicated by the condition of the studied children. These children can have serious cognitive and behavioural impairments from the underlying aetiology. Comparison of successful treatment with VGB to baseline is seriously complicated by positive effects on seizure outcome.

Lamotrigine (LTG)

The main antiepileptic mechanism of action is to block voltage-dependent sodium channels that result in prevention of excitatory neurotransmitter release (Meldrum, 1996). Clinical evidence indicates that LTG is effective in most seizure types, suggesting that other mechanisms might also play a role

The effect on cognition of LTG was compared to placebo in children with well-controlled or mild epilepsy in a double-blind, placebo-controlled, crossover study (Pressler et al., 2006). Forty-eight children with well-controlled or mild epilepsy were randomly assigned to add-on therapy either with LTG followed by placebo or placebo followed by LTG. Each treatment phase was nine weeks, with a crossover period of five weeks. No cognitive impairment was reported during active treatment compared with placebo.

Eun et al. (2012) compared monotherapy with LTG and CBZ in an open-label study of 84 children, of whom 67 (LTG 32 of 43, CBZ 35 of 41) completed the study. They reported that children treated with LTG did not differ statistically in intelligence from those treated with CBZ. There were no statistically significant differences between the two groups in terms of externalising behaviour but the parent report on the Conners scale showed an improvement ($p < 0.05$) in the CBZ group compared to the LTG group.

Buchanan (1995) studied the effects of LTG in a mixed group of children and adults with intellectual and physical disability, including 15 children (< 14 years of age). He reported that LTG resulted in marked cognitive improvement. Parental observations such as "marked improvement in alertness", "more part of the family" and "brighter and trying to walk" demonstrated a positive impact of LTG on aspects of patient quality of life. However, seizure control may have confounded these results.

The experiences of physicians and parents of 119 children on long-term LTG treatment was evaluated by conducting semi-structured interviews which assessed changes of cognition and vigilance (Brodbeck et al., 2006). The majority of patients, physicians and parents rated cognition and vigilance as unchanged during therapy. If changes were reported, these were more likely to be positive than negative for the patient and were most prominent in concentration and vigilance. Parent ratings were comparable to those of physicians.

The Rutter Behavioural Scales (parent version) were used by Fowler et al. (1994) to assess the behavioural effect in 47 children who were treated with LTG. Thirteen children passed from the disturbed to the non-disturbed range and only two patients went from the non-disturbed to the disturbed range.

Holmes et al. (2008) evaluated the effects on behaviour and psychosocial functioning of LTG monotherapy in children with newly-diagnosed typical absence seizures. Health outcome assessments included the Child Behaviour Checklist (CBCL) for ages 6-18, the Children's Global Assessment (C-GAS), and the Self-Perception Profile for Children (SPPC). These were completed at baseline screening and at the end of the maintenance phase. The CBCL showed an improvement in behaviour whereas the other measures were unchanged from baseline.

In conclusion, only a few studies reported adverse cognitive or behavioural effects and some evidence suggests that LTG has beneficial effects on behaviour, possibly through improved attention. However, seizure control may be a confounding factor.

Felbamate (FBM)

FBM was initially approved in 1993 for use as adjunctive therapy in the treatment of partial and generalized seizures associated with the Lennox-Gastaut syndrome in children. Following reports of aplastic anaemia and hepatic failure associated with FBM (French et al., 1999), its use was restricted to patients with severe epilepsy who had responded inadequately to other antiepileptic drugs. FBM is a broad-spectrum antiepileptic drug; it is a use-dependent sodium channel blocker and inhibitor of glutamate neurotransmission (Bialer et al., 2007).

No studies reporting the cognitive effects of FBM in children were found.

The behavioural effects of felbamate were assessed in 20 children aged two to 19 years with Lennox-Gastaut syndrome (Gay et al., 1995). Parents completed a questionnaire to evaluate behavioural change. Improvements were noted in social functioning, intellectual functioning, motor functioning, attention and concentration, alertness, initiative and variability in performance, and memory. After FBM was discontinued, parents again completed the same questionnaire. There was a tendency for these effects to reverse when the drug was discontinued. However, these positive findings were probably related to better seizure control.

In conclusion, there are no convincing data on the cognitive or behavioural effects of FBM.

Gabapentin (GBP)

The main mode of action of GBP appears to be through a selective inhibitory effect on voltage-gated calcium channels containing the $\alpha_2\delta$-1 subunit (Sills, 2006). It is used as second-line treatment for refractory partial seizures with or without secondary generalization.

No cognitive studies for children were found.

There are several paediatric reports of prominent behavioural change, including hyperactivity, irritability, and agitation (Khurana et al., 1996; Holmes, 1997; Morris, 1999). Mikati et al. (1998) compared twenty-six children with intellectual disability and six normal children, all with refractory partial seizures treated with add-on GBP. Behavioural adverse effects were more likely to occur in patients with intellectual disability in comparison with the intellectually normal group. Patients under 10 years of age, all of whom had intellectual disability, were more likely to have behavioural adverse effects than those who were over 10 years of age. These children had attention deficit disorder. Behavioural adverse effects resulted in discontinuation of the medication in only three patients.

Tallian et al. (1996) reported two children treated with GBP for refractory seizures who developed intolerable aggressive behaviour requiring dose reduction or drug discontinuation. Wolf et al. (1995) described three children with learning disability, one aged 7 years and two aged 10 years, with refractory partial seizures who developed severe behavioural problems while receiving GBP. The children became hyperactive and had explosive outbursts, consisting of aggressive and oppositional behaviour. The behavioural problems were sufficiently severe to require discontinuation of GBP. Lee et al. (1996) reported seven children who received GBP as adjunctive medication and developed behavioural adverse effects. Behaviours that parents considered most troublesome were tantrums, aggression directed toward others, hyperactivity and defiance. All behavioural changes were reversible and were managed by dose reduction or discontinuation of GBP. All children had baseline attention deficit hyperactivity disorder and developmental delay.

There is a suggestion that GBP may release or exacerbate pre-existing behavioural disturbances (Holmes, 1997). However, Besag (1996) did not confirm this in a study of 14 children and teenagers, most of whom had learning disability, treated with GBP for resistant epilepsy. The Rutter Behaviour parent scales indicated that two subjects moved from the non-disturbed range to the disturbed range and one moved from the disturbed range to the non-disturbed range. No differences were reported on the teacher scales. In a subsequent analysis with a control group, there were no differences in behaviour when GBP was added to the antiepileptic treatment.

In conclusion, there is no evidence for cognitive effects related to GBP. The evidence concerning behavioural effects is conflicting, with some studies indicating behavioural deterioration in children with pre-existing problems and one study revealing no such deterioration.

Topiramate (TPM)

TPM is a sulfamate-substituted monosaccharide with multiple mechanisms of action (White, 1997). It is licensed as monotherapy and adjunctive therapy.

Kang et al. (2007) evaluated the cognitive and behavioural effects of TPM and CBZ as monotherapy for children with benign Rolandic epilepsy. After 28 weeks of treatment, 88 children (45 on TPM and 43 on CBZ) were retested with a neuropsychological test battery. Two tests showed differences between the two treatments; arithmetic test scores decreased for TPM-treated children, compared with no change for CBZ-treated children, and the maze test showed more improvement for CBZ-treated children. Parents and teachers rated behaviour for the six-month baseline period and maintenance period for the 45 patients on TPM and 42 patients on CBZ, using the Conners Scales and the Child

Behavior Checklist. No significant changes were found but a larger change in the positive direction was found for the CBZ-treated patients and a negative trend for the TPM-treated patients.

Gerber et al. (2000) reported behavioural abnormalities in 11 of 75 (14.6%) children up to 18 years of age, between two weeks and four months after initiation of TPM therapy. They suggested that a previous history of behavioural problems and concurrent use of lamotrigine might be predisposing factors to behavioural disturbance.

Ness et al. (2012) reported the behavioural effects of adjunctive long-term TPM in 284 infants with a mean age of 12 months (standard deviation 6.3 months). On the Vineland Scales of Adaptive Behavior, a decline occurred in both the composite and domain standard scores from pre-treatment baseline to endpoint. However, individual domain raw scores increased, indicating that infants progressed in their acquisition of adaptive skill, but at a slower rate than the normative population.

The behavioural effects of TPM were also evaluated in children with intellectual disability in two studies. Coppola et al. (2008) added TPM to baseline antiepileptic medication in 29 children and adolescents, aged 3-19 years, with intellectual disability. At baseline, three months, six months, and 12 months, parents of all patients completed the Holmfrid Quality of Life Inventory. This inventory systematically evaluates the following domains: alertness, concentration, activation/tiredness, drowsiness, depression, aggressiveness and hyperactivity. Overall, TPM as an add-on drug caused mild to moderate behavioural worsening in about 70% of children and adolescents with mental retardation and epilepsy. This global worsening persisted after six (31%) and after 12 months follow-up (20%).

In another study, 16 adolescents with epilepsy and intellectual disability were assessed before and during treatment with TPM using the Rutter Behavioural Scales. There was a statistically significant increase in behavioural disturbances on both the parent and the teacher scales (Fowler et al., 1997).

In conclusion, in contrast to the studies on adults, only limited information exists on the cognitive effects of TPM in children. However, in view of the unequivocal cognitive adverse effects in adults, it is recommended that children who are treated with TPM should be monitored carefully for such effects. TPM can cause behavioural adverse effects, perhaps particularly in children and adolescents with intellectual disability, and these tend to persist over time, while they continue to take the drug.

Levetiracetam (LEV)

LEV is a broad-spectrum AED that has a novel proposed mode of action, namely binding to the synaptic vesicle protein SV2A (Lynch et al., 2004). It can be used as adjunctive therapy or monotherapy.

Levisohn et al. (2009) evaluated the neurocognitive effects of adjunctive LEV in children aged 4-16 years with inadequately-controlled partial-onset seizures. The results indicated that the effects on memory and attention, as measured by validated and well-standardized neurocognitive instruments, were no different from placebo over the eight to 12-week treatment period.

Schiemann-Delgado et al. (2012) investigated the cognitive and behavioural effects of adjunctive LEV in children aged 4-16 years with partial-onset seizures using the Leiter-R International Performance Scale and the Achenbach Child Behavior Checklist (CBCL).

Both tests showed an improvement from baseline at weeks 24 and 48. The authors concluded that, in children, adjunctive LEV was associated with long-term stability in cognitive functioning and improvement in behavioural functioning over time.

de la Loge et al. (2010) reported the effect of adjunctive LEV treatment on behavioural and emotional functioning using the Achenbach Child Behavior Checklist (CBCL) and the Child Health Questionnaire-Parent Form 50 (CHQ-PF50). Parents completed these questionnaires at baseline and after 12 weeks of treatment. The CBCL showed a worsening of aggressive behaviour in LEV-treated patients compared with improvement for placebo-treated patients, leading to similar results on the composite scores of externalizing syndromes and total problems. The CHQ-PF50 showed no differences.

Lagae et al. (2005) evaluated the effect of LEV in 77 children with a variety of childhood epilepsy syndromes with both partial and generalized seizures. A structured questionnaire was used to assess possible positive effects of LEV on alertness and behaviour. In 25% of the patients, a positive effect on alertness and/or behaviour was reported. Better alertness typically indicated better verbal or non-verbal communication between the caregivers and the child. Better behaviour in most children meant that the child could be handled and structured more readily. In most cases, the children were calmer.

A possible benefit of pyridoxine supplementation (vitamin B_6) in the treatment of LEV-induced behavioural adverse effects in a paediatric population has been suggested (Major et al., 2008).

In conclusion, existing studies do not demonstrate any substantial effect on cognition. In contrast, there is a suggestion of beneficial effects similar to LTG. The studies on behaviour show conflicting results but do not exclude the possibility of increased aggressiveness and hostility, as shown in adults.

Tiagabine (TGB)

TGB increases synaptic GABA by inhibiting its uptake into neurons and glia via inhibition of the GAT-1 GABA transporter, resulting in enhanced neuronal inhibition (Meldrum, 1996). It is approved by the U.S. Food and Drug Administration (FDA) as an adjunctive treatment for partial seizures in patients 12 years of age or older.

No published studies on the behavioural effects of TGB in children were found.

Oxcarbazepine (OXC)

OXC is a 10-keto analogue of CBZ. It is indicated as monotherapy or adjunctive therapy in patients with partial and secondarily generalised seizures.

Tzitiridou et al. (2005) studied 70 patients, aged 5-11 years, with newly-diagnosed benign childhood epilepsy with centrotemporal spikes, who were assigned to OXC monotherapy. Psychometric assessment was performed at baseline and after 18 months of treatment. No cognitive effects were demonstrated. Donati et al. (2006, 2007) investigated the effect of OXC on cognitive function in children aged 6-17 years with newly-diagnosed partial seizures in an open-label comparison with standard antiepileptic drug therapy (CBZ or VPA). Cognitive function and intelligence results for OXC did not differ from those of the other AEDs as monotherapy over a six-month treatment period. No impairment in cognitive function was observed in any treatment group over the six-month period.

There is one case report in German of a 15-year-old girl with tuberous sclerosis who developed rapid-cycling bipolar disorder when treated with OXC (Hagenah et al., 1999). However, tuberous sclerosis might represent a special case and no conclusions can be drawn from this single case report. More data are clearly needed.

In conclusion, OXC does not seem to induce negative cognitive effects. No data on behavioural effects were found.

Newest AEDs

Pregabalin (PGB)

As for GBP, the main mode of action of PGB appears to be through a selective inhibitory effect on voltage-gated calcium channels containing the $\alpha_2\delta$-1 subunit (Sills, 2006).

No studies on the cognitive or behavioural effects of PGB were found.

Stiripentol (STP)

No studies on the cognitive or behavioural effects of STP were found.

Rufinamide (RUF)

Rufinamide is a novel compound, structurally unrelated to other AEDs. The precise mechanism by which rufinamide exerts its anti-seizure effect is unknown. It can be used as adjunctive therapy in children and adults with Lennox-Gastaut syndrome and in adolescents and adults with partial seizures (Bialer et al., 2007).

No studies on the cognitive or behavioural effects of RUF were found.

Zonisamide (ZNS)

ZNS has multiple mechanisms of action, including calcium and sodium channel inhibition and carbonic anhydrase inhibition (Leppik, 2004). It can be used as adjunctive treatment in refractory partial seizures, with or without secondary generalized seizures in adults, and may be effective in Lennox-Gastaut syndrome, infantile spasms and progressive myoclonic epilepsy (Henry et al., 1988; Suzuki et al., 1997; Kyllerman and Ben-Menachem, 1998; Yanai et al., 1999; Lotze and Wilfong, 2004; You et al., 2008).

A lower dose of ZNS had more cognitive and behavioural benefits than a higher dose in children with newly diagnosed epilepsy (Eun et al., 2011). The Korean Wechsler Intelligence Scale for Children – Third edition (KWISC-III) was used for cognitive assessment and the Korean child behaviour checklist (K-CBCL) was used to measure behavioural problems. After 24 weeks of treatment with ZNS monotherapy, there was a cognitive worsening in the high-dose group but cognitive and behavioural improvement in the low-dose group. There was a lower cognitive score for the high-dose group than for the low-dose group and improvements were greater in the low-dose group than in the high-dose group.

ZNS has been used for many years in Japan and Korea but experience in other countries is very limited. There are a few case-reports, however, of behaviour disturbances provoked by ZNS monotherapy in children with epilepsy who are neither physically nor mentally disturbed. ZNS-induced behaviour disorders were reported in a 1-year-old girl and a 3-year-old boy (Kimura, 1994). Two of the 27 children with idiopathic epilepsy treated with ZNS monotherapy had behaviour disturbances which occurred several years later (Hirai et al., 2002). In one 14-year-old girl, selective mutism, violent behaviour and lack of concentration developed. In the other case, a 15-year-old girl, obsessive compulsive disorder (OCD) developed. Decreasing the dosage of ZNS reduced the problems.

Miyamoto et al. (2000) suggested that care should be taken in introducing ZNS in younger patients, particularly in children, because ZNS appeared to have contributed to psychotic episodes in two children. Furthermore, in children, obsessive-compulsive symptoms appeared to be related to psychotic episodes during ZNS treatment. However, little detailed information was provided.

In conclusion, limited information is available on ZNS. It is not possible to draw any firm conclusions with regard to the cognitive and behavioural effects of ZNS.

Lacosamide (LCS)

The molecular mechanisms of action of lacosamide have not yet been clarified. Lacosamide is approved as antiepileptic drug for patients 17 years or older with partial epilepsy by the US Food and Drug Administration.

There are sparse data on children. One study evaluated its use in 40 children with refractory epilepsy and a mean age of 14.3 years (Yorns et al., 2014). In most patients, lacosamide was added to the current medication and in four patients lacosamide was used as monotherapy. 37.5% had adverse effects and seven patients discontinued treatment. The reasons for discontinuation were because it was ineffective in improving seizure control in four patients and because of behavioural effects in only one patient. Another study, Ijff et al. (2015), showed cognitive-enhancing effects; however, this study was in adults.

Retigabine (RTG)

The primary mechanism of retigabine is through activation of KCNQ2 and KCNQ2/3 neuronal potassium channels. Secondary mechanisms of action include potentiation of GABA-evoked currents in cortical neurons via activation of $GABA_A$ receptors (Treven et al., 2015).

There is lack of systematic studies on the cognitive and behavioural effects of RTG in children.

Perampanel (PER)

Perampanel inhibits AMPA-induced increases in intracellular Ca^{2+} and selectively blocks AMPA receptor-mediated synaptic transmission, thus reducing neuronal excitation. The drug is approved for use in the European Union and United States (Shih et al., 2013).

Biro et al. (2015) carried out an observational, retrospective study of perampanel treatment on 58 young people, 2 to 17 years of age with refractory epilepsy. Behavioural changes (total $n = 14$, of which eight were aggression) were among the most frequent adverse effects.

Rosenfeld *et al.* (2015) examined the data on adolescents (12 to 17 years of age) treated with perampanel for refractory seizures in pooled, double-blind, placebo-controlled trials. One hundred and forty-three of the 1,480 patients were adolescents. Aggression was reported in 8.2%.

There is a suggestion that behavioural change, including aggression, might be dose-related but more data are required.

Recommendations

Based on this review of the existing data some very general recommendations can be provided. *Table 1* summarises these recommendations:

The bold typeface indicates evidence for adverse effects of antiepileptic drugs in children.

The first two columns provide AEDs that have shown negative cognitive or behavioural effects, whereas the last two columns give drugs for which there is evidence of positive effects on cognition and behaviour, respectively. The two neutral columns give drugs that have shown no cognitive or behavioural effects. The third column indicates that no data for children were found for 10 of the antiepileptic drugs; this lack of data is a cause for concern.

Acknowledgements

The extensive assistance of Dominique M. Ijff in the preparation of this manuscript is gratefully acknowledged.

Table 1. Recommendations for use of antiepileptic drugs in children, based on cognitive and behavioural complications

	Caution cognition[1]	Caution Behaviour[2]	Inconclusive/ lack of data	Neutral cognition[3]	Neutral behaviour[3]	Positive cognitive effects	Positive behavioural effects
Older AEDs	Phenobarbital Phenytoin	Phenobarbital Valproate	Ethosuximide Clobazam	Valproate Carbamazepine	Carbamazepine		
Newer AEDs	Topiramate	Gabapentin Topiramate Levetiracetam	Vigabatrin Felbamate Tiagabine	Gabapentin Oxcarbazepine		Lamotrigine Levetiracetam	Lamotrigine
Newest AEDs	Zonisamide	Zonisamide	Pregabalin Stiripentol Rufinamide Lacosamide Retigabine				

[1]. Caution cognition: sufficient data to recommend a careful monitoring of cognition in children because of the risk of potential cognitive adverse effects
[2]. Caution behaviour: sufficient data to recommend careful monitoring of behaviour in children because of the risk of potential behavioural adverse effects
[3]. Neutral: evidence exists for the absence of negative effects on either cognition or behaviour.

References

Aldenkamp AP, Alpherts WCJ, Blennow G, Elmqvist D, Heijbel J, Nilsson HL, et al. Withdrawal of antiepileptic medication in children – Effects on cognitive function: The multicenter Holmfrid study. Neurology 1993; 43(1): 41-50.

Bacon CJ, Cranage JD, Hierons AM, Rawlins MD, Webb JK. Behavioural effects of phenobarbitone and phenytoin in small children. Arch Dis Child 1981; 56(11): 836-40.

Bawden HN, Camfield CS, Camfield PR, Cunningham C, Darwish H, Dooley JM, et al. The cognitive and behavioural effects of clobazam and standard monotherapy are comparable. Canadian Study Group for Childhood Epilepsy. Epilepsy Res 1999; 33(2-3): 133-43.

Berg I, Butler A, Ellis M, Foster J. Psychiatric aspects of epilepsy in childhood treated with carbamazepine, phenytoin or sodium valproate: a random trial. Dev Med Child Neurol 1993; 35(2): 149-57.

Besag FMC. Gabapentin use with paediatric patients. Reviews in Contemporary Pharmacotherapy 1996; 7(5): 233-238.

Bialer M, Johannessen SI, Kupferberg HJ, Levy RH, Perucca E, Tomson T. Progress report on new antiepileptic drugs: a summary of the Eigth Eilat Conference (EILAT VIII). Epilepsy Res 2007; 73(1): 1-52.

Biro A, Stephani U, Tarallo T, Bast T, Schlachter K, Fleger M, et al. Effectiveness and tolerability of perampanel in children and adolescents with refractory epilepsies: first experiences. Neuropediatrics 2015; 46(2): 110-5.

Brodbeck V, Jansen V, Fietzek U, Muehe C, Weber G, Heinen F. Long-term profile of lamotrigine in 119 children with epilepsy. Eur J Paediatr Neurol 2006; 10(3): 135-41.

Broicher T, Seidenbecher T, Meuth P, Munsch T, Meuth SG, Kanyshkova T, et al. T-current related effects of antiepileptic drugs and a Ca2+ channel antagonist on thalamic relay and local circuit interneurons in a rat model of absence epilepsy. Neuropharmacology 2007; 53(3): 431-46.

Buchanan N. The efficacy of lamotrigine on seizure control in 34 children, adolescents and young adults with intellectual and physical disability. Seizure 1995; 4(3): 233-236.

Calandre EP, Dominguez-Granados R, Gomez-Rubio M, Molina-Font JA. Cognitive effects of long-term treatment with phenobarbital and valproic acid in school children. Acta Neurologica Scandinavica 1990; 81(6): 504-506.

Camfield CS, Chaplin S, Doyle AB, Shapiro SH, Cummings C, Camfield PR. Side effects of phenobarbital in toddlers; behavioral and cognitive aspects. J Pediatr 1979; 95(3): 361-5.

Coppola G, Verrotti A, Resicato G, Ferrarelli S, Auricchio G, Operto FF, et al. Topiramate in children and adolescents with epilepsy and mental retardation: a prospective study on behavior and cognitive effects. Epilepsy & Behavior 2008; 12(2): 253-256.

Darke K, Edwards SW, Hancock E, Johnson AL, Kennedy CR, Lux AL, et al. Developmental and epilepsy outcomes at age 4 years in the UKISS trial comparing hormonal treatments to vigabatrin for infantile spasms: a multi-centre randomised trial. Archives of Disease in Childhood 2010; 95(5): 382-386.

De La Loge C, Hunter SJ, Schiemann J, Yang H. Assessment of behavioral and emotional functioning using standardized instruments in children and adolescents with partial-onset seizures treated with adjunctive levetiracetam in a randomized, placebo-controlled trial. Epilepsy Behav 2010; 18(3): 291-8.

Donaldson GW, Graham JG. Aplastic anaemia following the administration of tegretol. Br J Clin Pract 1965; 19(12): 699-702.

Donati F, Gobbi G, Campistol J, Rapatz G, Daehler M, Sturm Y, et al. The cognitive effects of oxcarbazepine versus carbamazepine or valproate in newly diagnosed children with partial seizures. Seizure 2007; 16(8): 670-9.

Donati F, Gobbi G, Campistol J, Rapatz G, Daehler M, Sturm Y, et al. Effects of oxcarbazepine on cognitive function in children and adolescents with partial seizures. Neurology 2006; 67(4): 679-82.

Eke T, Talbot JF, Lawden MC. Severe persistent visual field constriction associated with vigabatrin. BMJ 1997; 314(7075): 180-181.

Eun SH, Eun BL, Lee JS, Hwang YS, Kim KJ, Lee YM, et al. Effects of lamotrigine on cognition and behavior compared to carbamazepine as monotherapy for children with partial epilepsy. Brain Dev 2012; 34(10): 818-23.

Eun SH, Kim HD, Eun BL, Lee IK, Chung HJ, Kim JS, et al. Comparative trial of low- and high-dose zonisamide as monotherapy for childhood epilepsy. Seizure 2011; 20(7): 558-63.

Farwell JR, Lee YJ, Hirtz DG, Sulzbacher SI, Ellenberg JH, Nelson KB. Phenobarbital for febrile seizures--effects on intelligence and on seizure recurrence. N Engl J Med 1990; 322(6): 364-9.

Ferrie CD, Robinson RO, Panayiotopoulos CP. Psychotic and severe behavioural reactions with vigabatrin: a review. Acta Neurologica Scandinavica 1996; 93(1): 1-8.

Forsythe I, Butler R, Berg I, Mcguire R. Cognitive impairment in new cases of epilepsy randomly associated to carbamazepine, phenytoin and sodium valproate. Developmental Medicine & Child Neurology 1991; 33(6): 524-534.

Fowler M, Besag FMC, Pool F. Effects of lamotrigine on behaviour in children. Epilepsia 1994; 35(Suppl 7): 69.

Fowler M, Besag FMC, Strange M, Pool F. Effects of topiramate on behaviour in adolescents with learning disability. Epilepsia 1997; 38(Suppl 3): 131.

French J, Smith M, Faught E, Brown L. Practice advisory: The use of felbamate in the treatment of patients with intractable epilepsy: report of the Quality Standards Subcommittee of the American Academy of Neurology and the American Epilepsy Society. Neurology 1999; 52(8): 1540-5.

Gastaut H. Preliminary trial of a benzodiazepine in epileptology. Nouv Presse Med 1978; 7(27): 2400.

Gay PE, Mecham GF, Coskey JS, Sadler T, Thompson JA. Behavioral effects of felbamate in childhood epileptic encephalopathy (Lennox-Gastaut syndrome). Psychological Reports 1995; 77(3 Pt 2): 1208-1210.

Gerber PE, Hamiwka L, Connolly MB, Farrell K. Factors associated with behavioral and cognitive abnormalities in children receiving topiramate. Pediatr Neurol 2000; 22(3): 200-3.

Glauser TA, Cnaan A, Shinnar S, Hirtz DG, Dlugos D, Masur D, et al. Ethosuximide, valproic acid, and lamotrigine in childhood absence epilepsy: initial monotherapy outcomes at 12 months. Epilepsia 2013; 54(1): 141-55.

Glauser TA, Cnaan A, Shinnar S, Hirtz DG, Dlugos D, Masur D, et al. Ethosuximide, valproic acid, and lamotrigine in childhood absence epilepsy. N Engl J Med 2010; 362(9): 790-9.

Hagenah U, Coners H, Kotlarek F, Herpertz-Dahlmann B. Tuberous sclerosis and organic bipolar disorder in a 15-year-old adolescent [German]. Zeitschrift Fur Kinder-Und Jugendpsychiatrie Und Psychotherapie 1999; 27(4): 283-289.

Henry TR, Leppik IE, Gumnit RJ, Jacobs M. Progressive myoclonus epilepsy treated with zonisamide. Neurology 1988; 38(6): 928-31.

Hirai K, Kimiya S, Tabata K, Seki T, Jozaki K, Kumagai N. Selective mutism and obsessive compulsive disorders associated with zonisamide. Seizure 2002; 11(7): 468-70.

Holmes GL. Gabapentin for treatment of epilepsy in children. Seminars in Pediatric Neurology 1997; 4(3): 244-250.

Holmes GL, Frank LM, Sheth RD, Philbrook B, Wooten JD, Vuong A, et al. Lamotrigine monotherapy for newly diagnosed typical absence seizures in children. Epilepsy Res 2008; 82(2-3): 124-32.

Ijff DM, Van Veenendaal TM, Majoie HJ, De Louw AJ, Jansen JF, Aldenkamp AP. Cognitive effects of lacosamide as adjunctive therapy in refractory epilepsy. Acta Neurol Scand 2015; 131(6): 347-54.

Jambaque I, Chiron C, Dumas C, Mumford J, Dulac O. Mental and behavioural outcome of infantile epilepsy treated by vigabatrin in tuberous sclerosis patients. Epilepsy Research 2000; 38: 151-160.

Jan MM, Shaabat AO. Clobazam for the treatment of intractable childhood epilepsy. *Neurosciences (Riyadh)* 2000; 5(3): 159-61.

Kalviainen R, Nousiainen I, Mantyjarvi M, Nikoskelainen E, Partanen J, Partanen K, et al. Vigabatrin, a gabaergic antiepileptic drug, causes concentric visual field defects. *Neurology* 1999; 53(5): 922-926.

Kang HC, Eun BL, Wu LC, Ku MH, Kim JS, Wook KD, et al. The effects on cognitive function and behavioral problems of topiramate compared to carbamazepine as monotherapy for children with benign rolandic epilepsy. *Epilepsia* 2007; 48(9): 1716-1723.

Khurana DS, Riviello J, Helmers S, Holmes G, Anderson J, Mikati MA. Efficacy of gabapentin therapy in children with refractory partial seizures. *Journal of Pediatrics* 1996; 128(6): 829-833.

Kimura S. Zonisamide-induced behavior disorder in two children. *Epilepsia* 1994; 35(2): 403-405.

Kumbier E, Haack K. Alfred Hauptmann – the fate of a german neurologist of jewish origin. *Fortschr Neurol Psychiatr* 2002; 70(4): 204-9.

Kwan P, Brodie MJ. Phenobarbital for the treatment of epilepsy in the 21st century: a critical review. *Epilepsia* 2004; 45(9): 1141-9.

Kyllerman M, Ben-Menachem E. Zonisamide for progressive myoclonus epilepsy: long-term observations in seven patients. *Epilepsy Res* 1998; 29(2): 109-14.

Lagae L, Buyse G, Ceulemans B. Clinical experience with levetiracetam in childhood epilepsy: an add-on and mono-therapy trial. *Seizure* 2005; 14(1): 66-71.

Lee DO, Steingard RJ, Cesena M, Helmers SL, Riviello JJ, Mikati MA. Behavioral side effects of gabapentin in children. *Epilepsia* 1996; 37(1): 87-90.

Leppik IE. Zonisamide: chemistry, mechanism of action, and pharmacokinetics. *Seizure* 2004; 13(Suppl 1): S5-S9.

Levisohn PM, Mintz M, Hunter SJ, Yang H, Jones J, Group NLS. Neurocognitive effects of adjunctive levetiracetam in children with partial-onset seizures: a randomized, double-blind, placebo-controlled, noninferiority trial. *Epilepsia* 2009; 50(11): 2377-89.

Loscher W. Basic pharmacology of valproate: a review after 35 years of clinical use for the treatment of epilepsy. *CNS Drugs* 2002; 16(10): 669-94.

Lotze TE, Wilfong AA. Zonisamide treatment for symptomatic infantile spasms. *Neurology* 2004; 62(2): 296-8.

Lux AL, Edwards SW, Hancock E, Johnson AL, Kennedy CR, Newton RW, et al. The United Kingdom Infantile Spasms Study (UKISS) comparing hormone treatment with vigabatrin on developmental and epilepsy outcomes to age 14 months: a multicentre randomised trial. *Lancet Neurology* 2005; 4(11): 712-717.

Lynch BA, Lambeng N, Nocka K, Kensel-Hammes P, Bajjalieh SM, Matagne A, et al. The synaptic vesicle protein SV2A is the binding site for the antiepileptic drug levetiracetam. *Proc Natl Acad Sci U S A* 2004; 101(26): 9861-6.

Major P, Greenberg E, Khan A, Thiele EA. Pyridoxine supplementation for the treatment of levetiracetam-induced behavior side effects in children: preliminary results. *Epilepsy & Behavior* 2008; 13(3): 557-559.

Marson AG, Kadir ZA, Hutton JL, Chadwick DW. The new antiepileptic drugs: a systematic review of their efficacy and tolerability. *Epilepsia* 1997; 38(8): 859-880.

Meldrum BS. Update on the mechanism of action of antiepileptic drugs. *Epilepsia* 1996; 37 Suppl 6: S4-11.

Mikati MA, Choueri R, Khurana DS, Riviello J, Helmers S, Holmes G. Gabapentin in the treatment of refractory partial epilepsy in children with intellectual disability. *Journal of Intellectual Disability Research* 1998; 42 Suppl 1: 57-62.

Mitchell WG, Chavez JM. Carbamazepine versus phenobarbital for partial onset seizures in children. *Epilepsia* 1987; 28(1): 56-60.

Miyamoto T, Kohsaka M, Koyama T. Psychotic episodes during zonisamide treatment. *Seizure* 2000; 9(1): 65-70.

Morris GL. Gabapentin. *Epilepsia* 1999; 40 Suppl 5: S63-S70.

Ness S, Todd MJ, Wang S, Eerdekens M, Nye JS, Ford L. Adaptive behavior outcomes in infants treated with adjunctive topiramate. *Pediatr Neurol* 2012; 46(6): 350-8.

O'callaghan FJ, Lux AL, Darke K, Edwards SW, Hancock E, Johnson AL, et al. The effect of lead time to treatment and of age of onset on developmental outcome at 4 years in infantile spasms: evidence from the United Kingdom Infantile Spasms Study. *Epilepsia* 2011; 52(7): 1359-1364.

Pal DK, Das T, Chaudhury G, Johnson AL, Neville BG. Randomised controlled trial to assess acceptability of phenobarbital for childhood epilepsy in rural India. *Lancet* 1998; 351(9095): 19-23.

Pressler RM, Binnie CD, Coleshill SG, Chorley GA, Robinson RO. Effect of lamotrigine on cognition in children with epilepsy. *Neurology* 2006; 66(10): 1495-9.

Riva D, Devoti M. Carbamazepine withdrawal in children with previous symptomatic partial epilepsy: effects on neuropsychologic function. *J Child Neurol* 1999; 14(6): 357-62.

Rosenfeld W, Conry J, Lagae L, Rozentals G, Yang H, Fain R, et al. Efficacy and safety of perampanel in adolescent patients with drug-resistant partial seizures in three double-blind, placebo-controlled, phase III randomized clinical studies and a combined extension study. *Eur J Paediatr Neurol* 2015.

Schain RJ, Ward JW, Guthrie D. Carbamazepine as an anticonvulsant in children. *Neurology* 1977; 27(5): 476-80.

Schiemann-Delgado J, Yang H, Loge Cde L, Stalvey TJ, Jones J, Legoff D, et al. A long-term open-label extension study assessing cognition and behavior, tolerability, safety, and efficacy of adjunctive levetiracetam in children aged 4 to 16 years with partial-onset seizures. *J Child Neurol* 2012; 27(1): 80-9.

Sheth RD, Goulden KJ, Ronen GM. Aggression in children treated with clobazam for epilepsy. *Clinical Neuropharmacology* 1994; 17(4): 332-337.

Shih JJ, Tatum WO, Rudzinski LA. New drug classes for the treatment of partial onset epilepsy: focus on perampanel. *Ther Clin Risk Manag* 2013; 9: 285-93.

Shorvon S. History of the Drug Treatment of Epilepsy Between 1955 and 1989 with Special Reference to the Role of the International League Against Epilepsy (ILAE). In: Shorvon S, Perucca E & Engel Jr. J (eds.) *The Treatment of Epilepsy*. Third ed. Chichester: Wiley, 2009: xxii-xxxviii.

Sills GJ. The mechanisms of action of gabapentin and pregabalin. *Current Opinion in Pharmacology* 2006; 6(1): 108-113.

Stores G, Williams P, Styles E, Zaiwalla Z. Psychological effects of sodium valproate and carbamazepine in epilepsy. *Archives of disease in childhood* 1992; 67(11): 1330-1337.

Sulzbacher S, Farwell JR, Temkin N, Lu AS, Hirtz DG. Late cognitive effects of early treatment with phenobarbital. *Clin Pediatr (Phila)* 1999; 38(7): 387-94.

Suzuki Y, Nagai T, Ono J, Imai K, Otani K, Tagawa T, et al. Zonisamide monotherapy in newly diagnosed infantile spasms. *Epilepsia* 1997; 38(9): 1035-8.

Tallian KB, Nahata MC, Lo W, Tsao CY. Gabapentin associated with aggressive behavior in pediatric patients with seizures. *Epilepsia* 1996; 37(5): 501-502.

Treven M, Koenig X, Assadpour E, Gantumur E, Meyer C, Hilber K, et al. The anticonvulsant retigabine is a subtype selective modulator of GABAA receptors. *Epilepsia* 2015; 56(4): 647-57.

Trimble MR, Cull C. Children of school age: the influence of antiepileptic drugs on behavior and intellect. *Epilepsia* 1988; 29 Suppl 3: S15-S19.

Tzitiridou M, Panou T, Ramantani G, Kambas A, Spyroglou K, Panteliadis C. Oxcarbazepine monotherapy in benign childhood epilepsy with centrotemporal spikes: a clinical and cognitive evaluation. *Epilepsy Behav* 2005; 7(3): 458-67.

Vining EP, Mellitis ED, Dorsen MM, Cataldo MF, Quaskey SA, Spielberg SP, et al. Psychologic and behavioral effects of antiepileptic drugs in children: a double-blind comparison between phenobarbital and valproic acid. *Pediatrics* 1987; 80(2): 165-74.

White HS. Clinical significance of animal seizure models and mechanism of action studies of potential antiepileptic drugs. *Epilepsia* 1997; 38 Suppl 1: S9-17.

Wolf SM, Forsythe A. Behavior disturbance, phenobarbital, and febrile seizures. *Pediatrics* 1978; 61(5): 728-31.

Wolf SM, Forsythe A, Stunden AA, Friedman R, Diamond H. Long-term effect of phenobarbital on cognitive function in children with febrile convulsions. *Pediatrics* 1981; 68(6): 820-3.

Wolf SM, Shinnar S, Kang H, Gil KB, Moshe SL. Gabapentin toxicity in children manifesting as behavioral changes. *Epilepsia* 1995; 36(12): 1203-1205.

Yanai S, Hanai T, Narazaki O. Treatment of infantile spasms with zonisamide. *Brain Dev* 1999; 21(3): 157-61.

Yorns WR, Jr., Khurana DS, Carvalho KS, Hardison HH, Legido A, Valencia I. Efficacy of lacosamide as adjunctive therapy in children with refractory epilepsy. *J Child Neurol* 2014; 29(1): 23-7.

You SJ, Kang HC, Kim HD, Lee HS, Ko TS. Clinical efficacy of zonisamide in Lennox-Gastaut syndrome: Korean multicentric experience. *Brain Dev* 2008; 30(4): 287-90.

Behavioural effects of epilepsy surgery

Frank Besag, Rochelle Caplan, Albert Aldenkamp,
David W. Dunn, Giuseppe Gobbi, Matti Sillanpää

Abstract

There are relatively few studies of the behavioural outcome of epilepsy surgery in children that have used standardised behavioural measures before and after the procedure. Those investigations that have used such measures are often on mixed groups with mixed pathology, implying that the numbers, when stratified, are very small. They are also often retrospective. Furthermore, because placebo surgery is generally not an option, the studies have been open and they are usually uncontrolled. The few available data suggest that, although individual children may benefit or deteriorate, there is little overall group effect of temporal or extratemporal surgery on behavioural/psychiatric outcome. Hemispherectomy has traditionally been associated with the expectation of marked behavioural improvement but firm data are lacking. Multiple subpial transection performed for electrical status epilepticus of slow-wave sleep in the Landau-Kleffner syndrome can result in marked improvements in cognition and behaviour. Vagus nerve stimulation appears to improve quality of life and mood/behaviour but again the quality of the data has been questioned. There is a need for large, prospective, multicentre, collaborative studies using standardised cognitive and behavioural measures before and after surgery to provide an adequate database on the outcome of various categories of procedures, pathologies and patients.

Key words: temporal, frontal, hemispherectomy, subpial transection, extratemporal, vagus nerve stimulation

In the past, the emphasis of antiepileptic treatment, both with medication and surgery, has been on seizure freedom. Over recent years the importance of outcome in terms of other measures, particularly with regard to cognitive and psychiatric issues, has also been recognised. Quality-of-life measures have been introduced before and after treatment to provide some indication of the overall success. This brief review will focus on the positive and negative behavioural/psychiatric effects of epilepsy surgery in children and teenagers. Each section will commence with the classical and/or larger studies.

■ Search strategy

Medline/PubMed was searched until March 2015 using the following terms: (child$ or pediat$ or adolescen$) and epilep$ and (behav$ or psychiat$ or psycho$) and (surg$ or lobectomy or hemispherectomy or resection or transection). The reference lists of key papers were checked for additional studies. Smaller initial studies that have subsequently been overtaken by larger or more comprehensive investigations have not been presented. Publications reporting mixed groups of patients undergoing different types of surgery with relatively small numbers in any subgroup have also not been reviewed here. The assistance of Professor Mary Lou Smith and Professor Helen Cross, in advising on relevant studies is also gratefully acknowledged.

■ Temporal lobe resection

Temporal lobe resection is the most frequently-performed neurosurgical procedure in adults with epilepsy. Much has been written on the psychiatric evaluation in this population. However, temporal lobe resections comprise only about 25% of epilepsy surgical procedures in children (Harvey et al., 2008) and there are few systematic studies of the psychiatric outcome of this procedure in this group.

A classical study on temporal lobe epilepsy in childhood was that of Lindsay et al. (1984) who followed 100 unselected children with between 1948 and 1982. Before surgery, the nine surviving patients who had undergone temporal lobectomy had a variety of major behavioural difficulties: four had been expelled from school or threatened with expulsion, three had near-suicidal depression, and four had been severely aggressive. They were followed to adulthood, when all were in regular work and none had any lasting psychiatric or social difficulties. The conclusion reached was that surgery could play a major beneficial role in selected cases of childhood temporal lobe epilepsy. A large and more recent study was that of McLellan et al. (2005), who carried out a case-note review on all the 62 children in the epilepsy surgery program at Great Ormond Street Hospital for Children, London, UK, who underwent temporal lobe surgery for medically-intractable epilepsy between 1992 and 1998. The case notes were reviewed independently by a paediatric neurologist and a child and adolescent psychiatrist. Particular note was taken of psychiatric assessments which had been carried out as part of the pre-operative and post-operative investigations. Two of the 62 children were excluded because they had Rasmussen encephalitis. Of the remaining 60 children, 35 were male and 25 were female. Seventy-one temporal lobe surgical procedures were performed. The mean age at first operation was 10 years 7 months (standard deviation 4 years 11 months, range seven months to 17 years 11 months). The mean age at seizure onset was 3.5 years. Thirty-three had hippocampal sclerosis, eight of whom had dual pathology. Twenty-three had a foreign tissue lesion. Six had cortical dysplasia/microdysgenesis. Six had other pathology. Cognitive ability was normal in 53% of the sample; of the remainder, 8% had mild intellectual disability, 22% had moderate intellectual disability and 17% had severe intellectual disability. The median number of seizures per month was 30 and the mean number of seizures per month was 98. Three children were lost to follow-up. Of the remainder, using the Engel (1993) classification, 60% had a class I outcome (seizure freedom), 5% class II (rare seizures), 16% class III (significant improvement in seizure control) and 19% class IV (no change or deterioration in seizure control). The percentage of subjects with specific psychiatric diagnoses before surgery and (in parenthesis) after surgery were as follows: pervasive developmental disorder 38% (37%), attention deficit hyperactivity disorder 23% (23%), oppositional defiant/conduct disorder 23% (23%), disruptive behaviour disorder – not otherwise specified 42% (44%), emotional disorder 8% (21%), eating disorder 2% (4%), conversion disorder 2% (2%) and psychosis 0% (2%). 83% had a diagnosis of a psychiatric disorder at any time: 72% (43/60) before surgery and 72% (41/57) after surgery. Some children acquired a diagnosis of psychiatric disorder and others no longer had a psychiatric disorder after surgery. Apart from emotional disorder, which appeared to be more frequent after surgery, there was very little change in the other diagnoses, with the exception of pervasive developmental disorder. In 23 subjects who had this diagnosis before surgery, two lost the diagnosis, 11 improved, in seven there was no change and three deteriorated. None developed this diagnosis as a result of the surgery. However, notwithstanding the improvement, the overall rate of pervasive developmental disorder diagnosis remained almost the same, namely 38% before the surgery and 37% after the surgery. With regard to predictors of psychiatric outcome, they found that there were generally no clear relationships between seizure freedom post-operatively and any psychopathology, although there was a suggestion that those who were seizure free were more likely to lose a DSM IV diagnosis (24%) than those who continued to have seizures (4%). However, in some of the children who were seizure free post-operatively, new psychiatric disorders emerged. The authors concluded that psychiatric assessment should form an integral part of the overall management and that both parents and children should have careful counselling about the possible mental health outcomes. It is, perhaps, worth adding that attention to post-surgical rehabilitation might also be worthwhile. Children who have had to live with seizures for many years might find it quite difficult, in some cases, to cope with seizure freedom and with the implications for added responsibility that this might bring, unless they have appropriate support and rehabilitation (Wilson et al., 2007).

One of the concerns that arises when considering any epilepsy neurosurgery is whether cognitive losses might cause more disadvantage than the ongoing seizures. The recent retrospective cohort study by Lah and Smith (2015) of 40 children who underwent temporal lobectomy for temporal lobe epilepsy indicated that this procedure was associated with a risk of only a mild fall in aspects of semantic memory, specifically naming and reading accuracy following left temporal lobectomy; other areas of memory and literacy were found to be unchanged. Similarly reassuring findings were reported by Lee et al. (2015) in a retrospective analysis of 20 children who underwent temporal lobectomy (eight dominant and 12 non-dominant). They concluded that temporal lobectomy in children did not produce a significant decline in intelligence or memory. Lendt et al. (1999) tested 20 children (10-16 years of age) before and three and 12 months after temporal lobe resections (10 right, 10 left). Overall memory performance did not change after surgery, with five children showing gains and four showing deterioration. Poor seizure control was linked to the memory deterioration. Language performance and attention improved significantly three months and one year after surgery, respectively.

Skirrow et al. (2011) carried out a long-term outcome study of temporal lobectomy in 42 children. The average post-operative follow-up period was nine years. 86% were seizure free and 57% were no longer taking antiepileptic medication. They reported a significant increase in IQ after a follow-up of more than five years, which was not found in a non-surgical comparison group. Psychosocial outcome, including quality of life was also better in the surgical group; these positive outcomes were more strongly associated with seizure freedom than with the surgery itself. These results emphasise the importance of a sufficiently long period of follow-up before decisions are made about the extent of any benefit of epilepsy neurosurgery.

Extratemporal focal surgery

The group at Great Ormond Street Hospital, London, also analysed the results of psychopathology in children before and after extratemporal surgery (Colonnelli et al., 2012). Of the 102 children who underwent focal resections outside the temporal lobe between 1997 and 2008, adequate data were available on 71. The median age of seizure onset was one year (range: birth to 12 years, mean 3 years, standard deviation 3 years). The mean age at surgery was 9 years (standard deviation 5 years). The majority of the resections were from the frontal lobe (73%). The remainder were parietal (17%) and occipital (10%). A detailed psychiatric assessment was carried out before surgery by an experienced child and adolescent psychiatrist. Post-operative psychiatric assessment was carried out one year after the surgery. Psychiatric diagnoses were based on the DSM IV classification. The rate of psychiatric diagnoses was remarkably similar preoperatively 31/77 (44%) and post-operatively 32/71 (45%). The psychiatric diagnoses included: ADHD, 6% preoperatively, 10% post-operatively, oppositional defiant disorder/conduct disorder, 13% preoperatively, 14% post-operatively, emotional disorder, 14% preoperatively and 17% post-operatively, autism spectrum disorder, 13% preoperatively and 14% post-operatively, disruptive disorder not otherwise specified, 20% preoperatively and 14% post-operatively. They pointed out that, within the category of disruptive behaviour disorder, 13% preoperatively and 9% post-operatively had a profile that was similar to the frontal lobe behaviour that is described in adults. The behaviour was characterised by one or more of the following features: disinhibition, emotional lability, unpredictability, lack of motivation, overactivity/underactivity.

Mental illness preoperatively was not associated with a worse surgical outcome in terms of seizure control. All children who had a new psychiatric diagnosis after surgery had undergone frontal lobe resection. The psychiatric deterioration did not appear to be related to poorer seizure control. They concluded, from their study, that frontal lobe pathology appeared to be related to a greater risk of psychopathology. In a commentary on this paper (Besag, 2012) it was pointed out that, although this was the largest published study of extra-temporal lobe epilepsy surgery in children, the numbers, when stratified, were quite small; there appears to be a great need for international collaboration, using standardised measures, to overcome the problem of small numbers in any one group.

In a more recent study, Andresen et al. (2014) presented results on 100 children, aged 6 to 16 years, who underwent temporal or frontal lobe surgery. The frontal lobe group had much poorer scores with regard to anhedonia and social concerns before the surgery than the temporal lobe group but there were marked improvements in the frontal group following the surgery. The changes with temporal lobe surgery were very much less. With regard to anhedonia, 63% of the frontal group improved, whereas 8% of the temporal lobe group improved. With regard to social concerns, 23% of the temporal lobe group improved whereas 100% of the frontal lobe group did so. With regard to aggressive behaviour, 3% of the temporal lobe group improved, compared with 9% who declined whereas 21% of the frontal lobe group improved and none declined.

There have been previous studies of children undergoing extra-temporal surgery but the overall numbers have tended to be quite small, implying that, when stratified, the numbers would have been even smaller.

■ Hemispherectomy

Although previous reviews of hemispherectomy, for example the early reviews carried out by Goodman (1986) and Lindsay (1987), and a number of subsequent papers (Beardsworth and Adams, 1988; Tinuper et al., 1988; Devlin et al., 2003; Lettori et al., 2008) reported a good behavioural outcome, established, standardised behavioural measures before and after surgery were generally not used. Devlin et al. (2003) studied the outcome of hemispherectomy in 33 children who had surgery from 0.33-17 years of age and had a median follow-up of 3.4 years (range: 1-8 years). As in most studies, there was a variety of pathology. They stated that behavioural improvement was reported in 92% of those who had preoperative behavioural problems. In one of the most recent studies, Althausen et al. (2013) carried out a questionnaire-based follow-up study on patients who had had various types of hemispherectomy surgery for a variety of pathologies. The total group was 81 patients, of whom questionnaires were returned for 61. All of the patients had at least one year follow-up with a mean follow-up period of 9.4 years (1.1-19.4). They divided the patients into three subgroups: early surgery, younger than 7 years at operation, intermediate surgery, 7-16 years at operation and late surgery, older than 16 years at operation. There were some striking differences between the groups, notably 90% seizure freedom in the early group, 73% in the intermediate group and 60% in the late group. The overall behavioural improvement ($N = 58$) was 57%, comprising 33% in the early group, 73% in the intermediate group and 61% in the late group. However, it must be noted that these results were based on retrospective evaluation through questionnaires and not on standardised measures before and after surgery. In contrast, Pulsifer et al. (2004) carried out a long-term neuropsychological follow-up study of 71 patients who underwent hemispherectomy; in this study, in addition to a number of cognitive measures, the authors used the Child Behaviour Checklist (CBCL) before and after the surgery. Twenty-five of the 71 (35%) were female. The group was almost equally divided between right and left hemispherectomies. The number with each underlying pathology and number who were seizure free (in parenthesis) were: Rasmussen encephalitis 37 (27), dysplasia 27 (12) and vascular 7 (7). With regard to quality-of-life measures, of the 41 patients who were able to respond, 20 (49%) rated their life in the past month as "most happy" and none rated their current life as "unhappy". For Rasmussen encephalitis, the overall CBCL result before surgery was 55.9 (standard deviation 9.9) and after surgery was 53.8 (standard deviation 13.8). For dysplasia, the overall CBCL result before surgery was 54.5 (standard deviation 9.3) and after surgery was 45.8 (standard deviation 9.1). For vascular aetiology, the overall CBCL result before surgery was 60.0 (standard deviation 8.9) and after surgery was 54.3 (standard deviation 17.7). These are not major changes. However, the authors pointed out that they did not find the extreme disturbance before surgery that had been reported in earlier studies, in which behaviours have been described as "serious outbursts of temper" and "gross behaviour disorder", including "murderous aggression". The cognitive improvements in the study carried out by Pulsifer et al. were described as "modest"; most of the IQ improvements were less than 15 points with only a few patients showing larger improvements.

Moosa et al. (2013) analysed the outcome of 115 hemispherectomy patients followed up for a mean of 12.7 years (range 2-28 years). On the basis of a simple structured outcome assessment, 54% had no behavioural problems and a further 19% had minimal behavioural problems with no impairment but no baseline behavioural data were provided. Seizure recurrence after hemispherectomy was the only factor predictive of poor behavioural outcome.

Functional hemispherectomy has also been performed on very young infants with severe epilepsy. Dorfer *et al.* (2015) reported four cases (three female, one male) of infants with "catastrophic epilepsy" who underwent functional hemispherectomy at 2.4 to 4.2 months of age. Three of the four were completely seizure-free after a median follow-up of 4.3 years (range 1.3 to 7.9 years). Performing presurgical and postsurgical behavioural measures on such young infants or comparing a surgical group with a control group would not be feasible/ethical but, in the light of information available on the behavioural outcome and, indeed, the survival of such infants who have not undergone surgery, it seems highly likely that the situation would have been improved by the surgery.

The consensus remains that hemispherectomy can improve behaviour to a considerable degree, although few studies have used standardised behavioural measures before and after surgery to confirm this. Families should be informed that no definitive predictions of outcome can be provided.

Multiple subpial transection

This procedure, developed by Frank Morrell (Morrell *et al.*, 1989), has mainly been used to treat children with ESES/CSWS, notably those with the Landau-Kleffner syndrome. Published data are very limited. Most case series do not report detailed behavioural outcomes, with the exception of the analysis carried out by Irwin *et al.* (2001). They presented data on nine children with the Landau-Kleffner syndrome (4 male, 5 female, age range 5.5-10 years). All the children had behavioural problems with inattention, hyperactivity and aggressive, oppositional behaviour that occurred in several settings. They were all either destructive and unmanageable or regressed and withdrawn. The authors coded six different domains with the score of 0, 1 or 2, to indicate whether the behaviour was normal, abnormal or severely abnormal, respectively. This implied that the most disturbed behaviour would have a score of 12. The pre-surgery scores ranged from 8 to 10. The post-surgery scores were initially 3 or 4 and, at the longest possible interval available following surgery, 1 (four of the five children) and 4 (the remaining child – the only one who required re-operation). They commented that the most striking effect of surgery was on behaviour. Following the surgery the children became interested in communicating. Attention span increased, hyperactivity resolved and the defiant aggressive behaviour disappeared.

Hypothalamic hamartoma

The classical presentation of a hypothalamic hamartoma is gelastic seizures, precocious puberty and behavioural problems. The behavioural problems can include outbursts of uncontrolled anger (Ng *et al.*, 2011). The epilepsy is typically resistant to medical treatment. Surgical treatment can result not only in seizure control but also improvement in behaviour (Ng *et al.*, 2006; Ng *et al.*, 2011). Ng *et al.* (2006) reported the results of transcallosal surgical resection in 26 patients, most of whom were children (mean age 10.0 years, range 2.1-24.2 years). Parents reported improvement in behaviour in 23 patients (88%) and improvement in cognition in 17 patients (65%). Standardised behavioural measures were not used, however. The same group also described a study of four patients (three male, one female) who underwent resection of hypothalamic hamartomas for behavioural indications. They reported striking improvements in the psychiatric comorbidity in all four subjects. One of these subjects was said to have been seizure-free before the surgery, again raising the question of whether subtle epileptic activity might have been playing a role, in this case affecting behaviour adversely before the surgery.

■ Vagus nerve stimulation

Studies on the possible psychiatric benefits of vagus nerve stimulation (VNS), mainly in adults, not necessarily with epilepsy, have indicated possible improvements in depression and anxiety disorders, including obsessive-compulsive disorder (O'Reardon et al., 2006; George et al., 2008). Several papers have reported improved quality of life with VNS, without providing specific behavioural measures. Mikati et al. (2009) examined the effects of the VNS in a mixed group of 16 patients, 11 of whom were children. Six had the Lennox-Gastaut syndrome. They found that seizure frequency reduction of more than 50% correlated with improvement in total quality of life ($p = 0.034$). Zamponi et al. (2011) examined the effect of VNS in 39 patients, 25 of whom had severe epilepsy with multiple independent spike foci and 14 of whom had the Lennox-Gastaut syndrome. They found that cognitive level and adaptive behaviour were unchanged but quality of life was improved in half of the patients.

A number of publications have reported behavioural improvement in children, although detailed behavioural data have generally not been presented. Parker et al. (1999) examined the outcome in all children who had insertion of a vagus nerve stimulator for epileptic encephalopathies in one centre over a two-year period. Sixteen children were included but the device was removed in one because of infection. They concluded that there were no significant improvements in seizure frequency or severity, nor was there any improvement in adaptive behaviour during the first year for the group as a whole but 4 children had "*a worthwhile reduction in seizure frequency*". Despite the lack of improvement in adaptive behaviour, they commented that there was an improvement in general behaviour. Majoie et al. (2001) compared the situation six months before vagus nerve implantation with six months after the surgery in children with a diagnosis of the Lennox-Gastaut syndrome. They reported a moderate improvement in mental functioning, behaviour and mood. The same group (Majoie et al., 2005) reported "*moderate improvement in functioning, behaviour and mood*" in 19 children with malignant childhood epilepsy resembling the Lennox-Gastaut syndrome treated with VNS at 24-month follow-up. They also commented that scores for mental age improved independently of the seizure control but this again raises the question of whether subtle manifestations of the epilepsy might have been ameliorated by an antiepileptic treatment.

Nagarajan et al. (2002) compared changes in quality of life, sleep and behaviour at last review with that prior to the VNS. The authors stated that, on a three-point scale, 12 of 16 children and adolescents with refractory epilepsy had improved quality of life with VNS and that this correlated with improved seizure control. Parental report indicated that behaviour was better in 12 children and worse in two. Sleep was said to be unchanged in 11 and improved in five. The authors reported that, in two children who had "*severe autistic traits*", a marked decrease in these traits occurred with VNS. This is in contrast to the findings of Danielsson et al. (2008) who, in a small, open prospective two-year follow-up study of eight children and adolescents with medically intractable epilepsy and autism, found no benefits of VNS on seizure frequency, cognition, autistic symptoms or behaviour. Kossoff and Pyzik (2004) reported dramatic improvement in aggression, social interaction and ambulation in three boys, aged 5-12 years with generalised slow spike-wave discharges and refractory epilepsy who were treated with a combination of topiramate and VNS. Hallböök et al. (2005b) examined the effect of VNS on cognitive ability, quality of life, behaviour and mood in 15 children with medically refractory epilepsy that were not eligible for epilepsy surgery. They used the Child Behaviour Checklist, Dodrill Mood Analogue Scale and the Birleson Depression Self-Rating Scale. A seizure frequency reduction of 50% or more was recorded in 6/15 of the children. Quality of life was improved in 13/15, of whom 11 also had improved seizure severity and mood; five, in addition, had an improvement in depressive parameters. The same group (Hallböök et al., 2005a) examined the sleep structure in these 15 children. 10 children had increased slow-wave sleep and of these, eight had improved quality of life. Eight were also said to have had improved behaviour.

Wilfong and Schultz (2006) reported the outcome of vagus nerve stimulation in seven girls (aged 1-14 years) with Rett syndrome and refractory epilepsy. At 12 months 6/7 had a seizure frequency reduction of 50% or more. Increased alertness was noted in all seven patients but there was no change in mood or communication ability. You et al. (2007) examined the effect of VNS in 28 children in Korea, using measures from the Korean version of the Quality of Life in Childhood Epilepsy questionnaire. They compared baseline with follow up of at least 12 months. There were improvements in memory in 9 (32%), mood in 12 (43%), behaviour in 11 (39.3%), alertness in 12 (43%), achievement in 6 (21.4%) and verbal skills in 8 (28.6%).

Reports of the positive effects of vagus nerve stimulation on psychiatric disorders have been questioned because most of the studies have been open and uncontrolled. It is possible to carry out controlled trials of vagus nerve stimulation by changing the stimulation parameters. There is a lack of such studies in evaluating the positive or negative behavioural consequences of vagus nerve stimulation in children.

■ Effect of timing of epilepsy surgery on outcome

Steinbok et al. (2009) identified 116 children who underwent epilepsy surgery in the first 3 years of life. The most common aetiologies were cortical dysplasia (34), tumour (22) and Sturge-Weber syndrome (19). Of the 107 patients in whom seizure outcome was assessed more than one year post-operatively, 72 (67.3%) were seizure free. Developmental information was available for 101 patients who had been followed up for more than one year. 16 of these were developmentally normal before and after surgery. Of the remaining 85, 47 (55.3%) were said to have improved in development compared to the preoperative situation, 28 showed no change and 10 were worse. However, formal neurodevelopmental assessments were completed before and after surgery in only 26 of these patients. In the whole group of 85 children there was a trend towards improvement in development in the 56 who became seizure free compared with those who continued to have seizures but the difference was not statistically significant ($p = 0.2$). The authors, nevertheless, concluded that early surgery may have a positive impact on development. Although no behavioural measures were reported, there is a strong link between developmental and behavioural outcomes, with the implication that if early surgery is associated with better developmental outcome it is also likely to be associated with better behavioural outcome. There is also a strong plausible argument for stating that the longer the child lives with having seizures, the more likely psychosocial impairment is to develop. This issue has been explored further by Lach *et al.* (2010), who carried out a study on the impact of paediatric epilepsy surgery on social inclusion in young adults. In the 38 patients who were seizure free in the previous 12 months, general social well-being was significantly better compared with those who were not seizure free (32 patients) and those who had not undergone surgery (31 patients). In a later study, the same group (Smith *et al.*, 2011) concluded that their results provided modest support for the suggestion that seizure freedom after paediatric surgery is associated with a reduced risk for psychological distress in early adulthood.

The same group (Elliott *et al.*, 2012) also found that seizure freedom after paediatric epilepsy surgery was associated with an improved quality of life in some domains. It is interesting to note that these results are in contrast to the short-term follow up study carried out by this group (Smith *et al.*, 2004) when they examined the cognitive, family function and psychosocial outcomes one year after paediatric epilepsy surgery and concluded that their findings challenged the assumption that seizure freedom resulted in an improvement in these domains, at least in the short-term. However, the two-year follow-up results suggested that improvement in social functioning might take time to develop after epilepsy surgery (Elliott *et al.*, 2008). Widjaja *et al.* (2011) evaluated the cost-effectiveness of paediatric epilepsy surgery compared to medical treatment. They concluded that it was a cost-effective treatment option in children with medically-refractory epilepsy but it is interesting to note that their model, while including costs associated with a number of factors, did not take account of several other issues, including psychosocial effects.

Basheer *et al.* (2007) examined the outcome of hemispheric surgery in children with refractory epilepsy. Twenty-four children with a variety of pathologies, including cortical dysplasia, infarction, Sturge-Weber syndrome and Rasmussen encephalitis were included. They stated that poor adaptive function was associated with a longer duration of epilepsy, older age at time of surgery and a history of infantile spasms. They also concluded that early age at surgery was associated with better adaptive outcome.

■ Conclusions

The spectrum of children coming to epilepsy surgery is wide. The rate of psychiatric disorder in this group is high and the benefits of surgery remain difficult to assess. The behavioural outcome following both temporal and extratemporal epilepsy neurosurgery in children is very variable, with some children improving and others deteriorating. Early surgical intervention and postoperative seizure freedom are associated with a better adaptive outcome. The outlook for hemispherectomy in behavioural terms appears to be somewhat better than for other procedures, although extensive data to confirm this impression remains elusive. There is a strong argument for ensuring that multicentre prospective data are collected on all forms of epilepsy neurosurgery in children so that adequate numbers can be obtained to allow a meaningful statistical analysis, even after stratification into the various subgroups according to age, gender, type of pathology and other key variables. Collection of such data might allow more accurate prognostic predictions for the behavioural outcome of epilepsy neurosurgery in the future.

References

Althausen A, Gleissner U, Hoppe C, Sassen R, Buddewig S, von LM, et al. Long-term outcome of hemispheric surgery at different ages in 61 epilepsy patients. *J.Neurol.Neurosurg.Psychiatry* 2013; 84(5): 529-536.

Andresen EN, Ramirez MJ, Kim KH, Dorfman AB, Haut JS, Klaas PA, et al. Effects of surgical side and site on mood and behavior outcome in children with pharmacoresistant epilepsy. *Front Neurol* 2014; 5: 18.

Basheer SN, Connolly MB, Lautzenhiser A, Sherman EM, Hendson G, Steinbok P. Hemispheric surgery in children with refractory epilepsy: seizure outcome, complications, and adaptive function. *Epilepsia* 2007; 48(1): 133-140.

Beardsworth ED, Adams CB. Modified hemispherectomy for epilepsy: early results in 10 cases. *Br.J.Neurosurg.* 1988; 2(1): 73-84.

Besag FMC. Psychopathological outcome of extratemporal lobe surgery: the need for international collaboration on data collection. *Dev.Med.Child Neurol.* 2012; 54(6): 486.

Colonnelli MC, Cross JH, Davies S, D'Argenzio L, Scott RC, Pickles A, et al. Psychopathology in children before and after surgery for extratemporal lobe epilepsy. *Developmental Medicine and Child Neurology* 2012; 54(6): 521-526.

Danielsson S, Viggedal G, Gillberg C, Olsson I. Lack of effects of vagus nerve stimulation on drug-resistant epilepsy in eight pediatric patients with autism spectrum disorders: a prospective 2-year follow-up study. *Epilepsy Behav.* 2008; 12(2): 298-304.

Devlin A, Cross J, Harkness W, Chong W, Harding B, Vargha-Khadem F, et al. Clinical outcomes of hemispherectomy for epilepsy in childhood and adolescence. *Brain* 2003; 126(3): 556-566.

Dorfer C, Ochi A, Snead OC, 3rd, Donner E, Holowka S, Widjaja E, et al. Functional hemispherectomy for catastrophic epilepsy in very young infants: technical considerations and complication avoidance. *Childs Nerv Syst* 2015.

Elliott I, Kadis DS, Lach L, Olds J, McCleary L, Whiting S, et al. Quality of life in young adults who underwent resective surgery for epilepsy in childhood. *Epilepsia* 2012; 53(9): 1577-1586.

Elliott IM, Lach L, Kadis DS, Smith ML. Psychosocial outcomes in children two years after epilepsy surgery: has anything changed? *Epilepsia* 2008; 49(4): 634-641.

Engel Jr. J, Van Ness PC, Rasmussen TB, Ojemann LM. Outcome with respect to epileptic seizures. In: Engel Jr. J (ed.) *Surgical treatment of the epilepsies*. New York: Raven Press, 1993: 609-621.

George MS, Ward HE, Jr., Ninan PT, Pollack M, Nahas Z, Anderson B, et al. A pilot study of vagus nerve stimulation (VNS) for treatment-resistant anxiety disorders. *Brain Stimulation* 2008; 1(2): 112-121.

Goodman R. Hemispherectomy and its alternatives in the treatment of intractable epilepsy in patients with infantile hemiplegia. *Developmental Medicine & Child Neurology* 1986; 28(2): 251-258.

Hallböök T, Lundgren J, Köhler S, Blennow G, Strömblad L, Rosén I. Beneficial effects on sleep of vagus nerve stimulation in children with therapy resistant epilepsy. *European Journal of Paediatric Neurology* 2005a; 9(6): 399-407.

Hallböök T, Lundgren J, Stjernqvist K, Blennow G, Strömblad LG, Rosén I. Vagus nerve stimulation in 15 children with therapy resistant epilepsy; its impact on cognition, quality of life, behaviour and mood. *Seizure* 2005b; 14(7): 504-513.

Harvey AS, Cross JH, Shinnar S, Mathern GW. Defining the spectrum of international practice in pediatric epilepsy surgery patients. *Epilepsia* 2008; 49(1): 146-155.

Kossoff EH, Pyzik PL. Improvement in alertness and behavior in children treated with combination topiramate and vagus nerve stimulation. *Epilepsy & Behavior* 2004; 5(2): 256-259.

Lach LM, Elliott I, Giecko T, Olds J, Snyder T, McCleary L, et al. Patient-reported outcome of pediatric epilepsy surgery: social inclusion or exclusion as young adults? *Epilepsia* 2010; 51(10): 2089-2097.

Lah S, Smith ML. Verbal memory and literacy outcomes one year after pediatric temporal lobectomy: a retrospective cohort study. *Epilepsy Behav* 2015; 44: 225-33.

Lee YJ, Kang HC, Kim HD, Kim DS, Shim KW, Eom S, et al. Neurocognitive function in children after anterior temporal lobectomy with amygdalohippocampectomy. *Pediatr Neurol* 2015; 52(1): 88-93.

Lendt M, Helmstaedter C, Elger CE. Pre- and postoperative neuropsychological profiles in children and adolescents with temporal lobe epilepsy. *Epilepsia* 1999; 40(11): 1543-1550.

Lettori D, Battaglia D, Sacco A, Veredice C, Chieffo D, Massimi L, et al. Early hemispherectomy in catastrophic epilepsy: a neuro-cognitive and epileptic long-term follow-up. *Seizure* 2008; 17(1): 49-63.

Lindsay J, Ounsted C, Richards P. Hemispherectomy for childhood epilepsy: a 36-year study. *Developmental Medicine & Child Neurology* 1987; 29(5): 592-600.

Lindsay J, Ounsted C, Richards P. Long-term outcome in children with temporal lobe seizures. V: Indications and contra-indications for neurosurgery. *Developmental Medicine & Child Neurology* 1984; 26(1): 25-32.

Majoie HJ, Berfelo MW, Aldenkamp AP, Evers SM, Kessels AG, Renier WO. Vagus nerve stimulation in children with therapy-resistant epilepsy diagnosed as Lennox-Gastaut syndrome: clinical results, neuropsychological effects, and cost-effectiveness. *Journal of Clinical Neurophysiology* 2001; 18(5): 419-428.

Majoie HJ, Berfelo MW, Aldenkamp AP, Renier WO, Kessels AG. Vagus nerve stimulation in patients with catastrophic childhood epilepsy, a 2-year follow-up study. *Seizure* 2005; 14(1): 10-18.

McLellan A, Davies S, Heyman I, Harding B, Harkness W, Taylor D, et al. Psychopathology in children with epilepsy before and after temporal lobe resection. *Dev.Med.Child Neurol.* 2005; 47(10): 666-672.

Mikati MA, Ataya NF, El-Ferezli JC, Baghdadi TS, Turkmani AH, Comair YG, et al. Quality of life after vagal nerve stimulator insertion. *Epileptic Disorders* 2009; 11(1): 67-74.

Moosa AN, Jehi L, Marashly A, Cosmo G, Lachhwani D, Wyllie E, et al. Long-term functional outcomes and their predictors after hemispherectomy in 115 children. *Epilepsia* 2013; 54(10): 1771-9.

Morrell F, Whisler WW, Bleck TP. Multiple subpial transection: A new approach to the surgical treatment of focal epilepsy. *Journal of Neurosurgery* 1989; 70(2): 231-239.

Nagarajan L, Walsh P, Gregory P, Lee M. VNS therapy in clinical practice in children with refractory epilepsy. *Acta Neurologica Scandinavica* 2002; 105(1): 13-17.

Ng YT, Hastriter EV, Wethe J, Chapman KE, Prenger EC, Prigatano GP, et al. Surgical resection of hypothalamic hamartomas for severe behavioral symptoms. *Epilepsy Behav* 2011; 20(1): 75-8.

Ng YT, Rekate HL, Prenger EC, Chung SS, Feiz-Erfan I, Wang NC, et al. Transcallosal resection of hypothalamic hamartoma for intractable epilepsy. *Epilepsia* 2006; 47(7): 1192-202.

O'Reardon JP, Cristancho P, Peshek AD. Vagus Nerve Stimulation (VNS) and Treatment of Depression: To the Brainstem and Beyond. *Psychiatry (Edgmont.)* 2006; 3(5): 54-63.

Parker AP, Polkey CE, Binnie CD, Madigan C, Ferrie CD, Robinson RO. Vagal nerve stimulation in epileptic encephalopathies. *Pediatrics* 1999; 103(4:Pt 1): t-82.

Pulsifer MB, Brandt J, Salorio CF, Vining EP, Carson BS, Freeman JM. The cognitive outcome of hemispherectomy in 71 children. *Epilepsia* 2004; 45(3): 243-254.

Skirrow C, Cross JH, Cormack F, Harkness W, Vargha-Khadem F, Baldeweg T. Long-term intellectual outcome after temporal lobe surgery in childhood. *Neurology* 2011; 76(15): 1330-1337.

Smith ML, Elliott IM, Lach L. Cognitive, psychosocial, and family function one year after pediatric epilepsy surgery. *Epilepsia* 2004; 45(6): 650-660.

Smith ML, Kelly K, Kadis DS, Elliott IM, Olds J, Whiting S, et al. Self-reported symptoms of psychological well-being in young adults who underwent resective epilepsy surgery in childhood. *Epilepsia* 2011; 52(5): 891-899.

Steinbok P, Gan PY, Connolly MB, Carmant L, Barry SD, Rutka J, et al. Epilepsy surgery in the first 3 years of life: a Canadian survey. *Epilepsia* 2009; 50(6): 1442-1449.

Tinuper P, Andermann F, Villemure JG, Rasmussen TB, Quesney LF. Functional hemispherectomy for treatment of epilepsy associated with hemiplegia: rationale, indications, results, and comparison with callosotomy. *Ann.Neurol.* 1988; 24(1): 27-34.

Widjaja E, Li B, Schinkel CD, Puchalski RL, Weaver J, Snead OC, et al. Cost-effectiveness of pediatric epilepsy surgery compared to medical treatment in children with intractable epilepsy. *Epilepsy Res.* 2011; 94(1-2): 61-68.

Wilfong AA, Schultz RJ. Vagus nerve stimulation for treatment of epilepsy in Rett syndrome. *Developmental Medicine & Child Neurology* 2006; 48(8): 683-686.

Wilson SJ, Bladin PF, Saling MM. The burden of normality: a framework for rehabilitation after epilepsy surgery. *Epilepsia* 2007; 48 Suppl 9: 13-16.

You SJ, Kang HC, Kim HD, Ko TS, Kim DS, Hwang YS, et al. Vagus nerve stimulation in intractable childhood epilepsy: a Korean multicenter experience. *Journal of Korean Medical Science* 2007; 22(3): 442-445.

Zamponi N, Passamonti C, Cesaroni E, Trignani R, Rychlicki F. Effectiveness of vagal nerve stimulation (VNS) in patients with drop-attacks and different epileptic syndromes. *Seizure* 2011; 20(6): 468-474.

When should pharmacotherapy for psychiatric/behavioural disorders in children with epilepsy be prescribed?

Frank Besag, Albert Aldenkamp, Rochelle Caplan, David W. Dunn, Giuseppe Gobbi, Matti Sillanpää

Abstract

The most important factor in deciding whether psychotropic medication should be prescribed is a meticulous assessment of the possible causes of the behavioural/psychiatric disturbance. This assessment should include a consideration of the possible roles of the epilepsy itself, treatment of the epilepsy, associated brain damage or dysfunction, reactions to the epilepsy and causes that are unrelated to the epilepsy or its treatment. If the epilepsy itself or antiepileptic drug treatment are responsible for the disorder then a review of antiepileptic medication is required. Contrary to popular myth, most psychotropic medications are not contraindicated in children with epilepsy. Treatment with methylphenidate, dexamfetamine, atomoxetine, clonidine or low-dose risperidone are unlikely to precipitate seizures. The selective serotonin reuptake inhibitors might protect against seizures but some of these are powerful enzyme inhibitors, implying that careful monitoring to avoid antiepileptic drug toxicity is recommended. In many cases, the appropriate approach will be through other interventions such as behavioural management or providing the young person with empowering strategies, implying that psychotropic pharmacotherapy should not be the first-line treatment. However, if assessment indicates that psychotropic medication is necessary, it can be of great benefit.

Key words: postictal, absence, CSWS, anxiety, depression

Before considering pharmacotherapy, the first step must be to assess the situation meticulously to determine the cause or causes of the disorder. There are several situations in which epilepsy-related behavioural disturbance occurs when it is inappropriate to prescribe psychotropic medication (Besag, 2002b). A systematic approach is recommended, to enable the clinician to make a rational decision about when to prescribe psychotropic medication and when to avoid doing so. Broadly speaking, the categories can be subdivided as follows (Besag, 2002a).

1. The epilepsy itself.
2. Treatment of the epilepsy.
3. Reactions to the epilepsy.
4. Associated brain damage/dysfunction.
5. Causes also applicable to those who do not have epilepsy.

Some of the psychiatric disorders that occur in children with epilepsy could fall into more than one of these categories, emphasising the importance of carrying out a careful assessment. For example, a child with the features of ADHD might have these as a result of inappropriate antiepileptic medication such as a phenobarbital (Wolf and Forsythe, 1978) or as a result of frequent absence seizures (Kaufmann et al., 2009). Psychosis could be related to the epilepsy (category 1 above) (Kanemoto et al., 1996), precipitated by an antiepileptic drug, such as vigabatrin or topiramate, (category 2) (Besag, 2001) or it could fall into the category of causes also applicable to those without epilepsy (category 5). The management of a postictal psychosis, a drug-induced psychosis or a "functional psychosis" would all be very different.

The indications for pharmacotherapy and other forms of management relating to each individual category will now be discussed.

■ Search strategy

In addition to papers already known to the authors, including those discussed earlier in this volume, the Medline/PubMed database was searched from inception until the end of March 2015 using the search terms: epilep$ and (child$ or adolescen$) and (behav$ or psychiat$) and treatment. Abstracts of likely relevance to the topic were examined to select papers for final detailed review. Reference lists of included papers were searched for any further relevant studies.

■ The epilepsy itself

Prodrome

Prodrome is that period, typically lasting from about half an hour to two days, sometimes longer, before a seizure or cluster of seizures, during which mood and consequently behaviour may be disturbed (Rajna et al., 1997). When the seizure occurs, the prodrome is terminated. Parents often recognise prodrome but there may be years of delay before any professional informs them that this is part of the epilepsy and not simply the child being "naughty". This information can be very valuable and empowering for families. There is no established pharmacotherapy for treating prodrome but if the seizures are completely controlled then the prodromes should also resolve. There are two, as yet unproven, possible consequences of antiepileptic therapy relating to prodrome that are worthy of discussion, although they are seldom mentioned. The first is that it is possible for a child with well-established prodromes, occasionally to have a prodrome without the following seizure. At first this might seem like a contradiction in terms. However, if the child goes through the usual sequence of the prodrome heralding the seizure but, just before the seizure is due to occur, some factor comes into operation raising the seizure threshold to such an extent that the seizure does not occur, this does not negate the fact that the phenomenon of the prodrome has occurred. It is not uncommon for families to describe the situation of a child who has regular prodromes followed by seizures but occasionally has a prodrome that is not followed by a seizure. The second situation that is seldom discussed is the possibility that the prodromes might become worse when seizures are partly controlled. The usual sequence of events is that each prodrome resolves with the ensuing seizure; however, if the seizure threshold is raised so the prodrome still occurs but the seizure does not, then the possibility arises that the prodrome might be more prolonged, *i.e.* it is not terminated by the seizure as soon as usual. If this situation were to occur, it might be tempting to decrease the antiepileptic medication to allow the seizures to return. However, there might, on the contrary, be a case for more effective antiepileptic treatment rather than less effective antiepileptic treatment, the aim being not only to prevent the seizures but also to prevent the prodromes.

It is not unusual to find parents stating that the prescription of an antiepileptic drug has improved seizure control but has also led to a deterioration in behaviour. There are several possible causes for this (also see later) but one possibility, particularly in a child with a history of prodrome, might be the situation just described. There appear to be no data, however, to show whether increasing antiepileptic medication rather than decreasing it improves the behaviour in such circumstances.

Aura

The aura is sometimes described as being the warning of the seizure. An aura is actually a focal seizure without impairment of awareness (simple partial seizure) and is, consequently, not a "warning" but actually the beginning of the seizure, before the epileptic activity has spread further into the brain. Typical auras include unpleasant sensations in the upper abdomen (the epigastric aura) or the head (the cephalic aura). However, auras can be experienced in almost any part of the body or can affect a variety of the senses (*e.g.* olfactory, visual), depending on the location of the epileptiform discharge that is giving rise to the apparent sensation. Some auras manifest as indescribably unpleasant feelings: dysphoric auras. Classical studies in adults, including that of Lennox and Cobb (1933), have indicated that auras are rarely pleasant and most of them are unpleasant. One of the most common auras is the epigastric aura (Gupta *et al.*, 1983).

In some patients, multiple auras can occur in a single day. This can be very distressing. Because the unpleasant aura raises anxiety, a vicious circle may develop, with the aura causing anxiety, lowering seizure threshold, making the next aura more likely to occur, and so on, repeatedly. An effective way to break into this vicious circle is to treat with an oral benzodiazepine, prescribed not as an anxiolytic drug but as an antiepileptic drug. This can resolve the situation in a short period of time: as long as it takes for the benzodiazepine to become absorbed into the bloodstream and effective in the brain. With the advent of buccal midazolam (Scott *et al.*, 1999; Mcintyre *et al.*, 2005), this mode of treatment could be considered for rapid control of repeated auras, if they are particularly distressing.

Automatism

Automatism might be defined as an action that does not appear to arise out of the will. In this sense, it is "automatic". Automatisms commonly occur in association with complex partial (dyscognitive) seizures (Fenton, 1975). Automatisms can also occur in the postictal phase. Some automatisms may be misinterpreted as aggressive behaviour. For example, automatisms in association with frontal lobe seizures may involve the flinging about of a single limb or cycling movements of the lower limbs (Scheffer et al., 1995). If a carer happens to be in the way of the moving limbs, the patient may gain a reputation of being someone who hits or kicks people. This could be misinterpreted as very violent, wilful behaviour when, on the contrary, it is totally involuntary. The importance of meticulous history-taking cannot be over-emphasised in such cases.

The key questions to ask in such a situation are as follows.

First, was the person fully aware? Awareness is usually impaired in the automatisms of complex partial (dyscognitive) seizures (Fenton, 1975).

Second, was the violence directed or was it simply the result of someone happening to be in the way? Automatisms do not usually consist of directed behaviour (Treiman, 1986).

Third, did the person recall what they had done afterwards? Automatisms are not usually recalled (Fenton, 1975).

In terms of the pharmacotherapy of automatisms, again, there is no specific psychotropic medication that is recommended because the aim should be to achieve better overall seizure control by optimising the antiepileptic medication or, if appropriate, referring the subject for epilepsy neurosurgery.

Postictal changes

One of the most common postictal changes is tiredness (fatigue) (Kanner et al., 2004), which can be associated with irritability. It is not unusual for patients to be confused after a seizure and, in their confusion, they may misinterpret an individual who has come to help them as someone coming to harm them, pushing them away, possibly violently (Treiman, 1986). Disinhibition can also occur after a seizure; if the seizure has involved the frontal lobes, the disinhibition can be marked. Again, this can cause much confusion. If, for example, the doctor or nurse witnesses postictal disinhibited behaviour they may, quite correctly, state that this is not an epileptic seizure. If they have not been aware of the preceding seizure, they might even interpret this behaviour as being unrelated to the epilepsy when, in fact, it is very much related to the preceding seizure and represents the period of recovery following the seizure, the postictal recovery period.

Postictal mood changes can also occur (Kanner et al., 2004). The patient may become elevated in mood or become depressed after a seizure or cluster of seizures. Pharmacotherapy is not usually appropriate for postictal depression; the depression will usually have resolved before antidepressant medication would have had time to become effective. Postictal elevated mood is usually relatively mild and does not require treatment. If severe postictal elevated mood, potentially placing the patient or others at risk, were to occur then the prescription of standard treatment for acutely elevated mood, such as olanzapine, might be appropriate.

Postictal paranoid schizophreniform psychosis can occur, typically after a cluster of seizures, in susceptible individuals (*Epilepsy and psychosis in children and teenager*, p. XX-XX). Depending on severity, this may require treatment. Postictal psychosis is well documented in adults (Kanemoto et al., 1996) but can also occur in teenagers. The duration is typically up to a few weeks. The postictal psychosis may recur after subsequent clusters of seizures. If the psychosis is distressing or is associated with risk, either to the individual or to others, then treatment with neuroleptic medication, such as risperidone, should be considered and may be appropriate. This is sometimes withheld because of a mistaken belief that there is a high risk of precipitating further seizures. Serious seizure exacerbations are unlikely to occur with the current atypical antipsychotic drugs prescribed in the usual doses (Pisani et al., 2002). The exception is clozapine (Devinsky et al., 1991), which would not usually be prescribed in this situation because it is reserved for resistant psychosis; however, it should be noted that there is good evidence to indicate that the seizure risk with clozapine is dose/blood-level related (Varma et al., 2011), implying that low doses might not be associated with a high risk. Withdrawing the antipsychotic treatment slowly once the psychotic symptoms have resolved, and monitoring closely for any recurrence of the psychotic symptoms, is a reasonable course of action although, as already stated, further treatment may be required after subsequent clusters of seizures.

Interictal psychoses

These may be schizophreniform or affective, although more commonly schizophreniform psychosis is reported (Kanemoto et al., 1996).

The term interictal psychosis, as currently used, covers two very different situations (*Epilepsy and psychosis in children and teenager*, p. XX-XX). Strictly speaking, the term should refer to a psychosis that occurs between seizures but has no clear time relationship to them. This type of interictal psychosis can certainly occur in teenagers with epilepsy. As is the case for postictal psychosis, if the psychosis is causing distress or is associated with significant risk, then treatment with neuroleptic medication will probably be indicated. This may need to be continued for much longer periods than is the case for postictal psychoses, however. The second situation covered by the term interictal psychosis probably should correctly be termed "post-epilepsy psychosis" because the onset of the psychosis is usually years after the seizures have ceased to occur. The interval between the resolution of the epilepsy and the onset of the psychosis is typically at least a decade. Again, consideration would be given to treating a schizophreniform psychosis with neuroleptic medication if the indications already discussed applied. If such indications applied to an affective psychosis then treatment with a mood-levelling antiepileptic drug such as sodium valproate or carbamazepine might be indicated, although in some instances neuroleptic medication may also be prescribed if more rapid mood stabilisation is required. This type of psychosis can be recurrent.

Focal epileptiform discharges

Temporal lobe epilepsy with onset in childhood can be associated with aggression which, in classical research, was said to respond to temporal lobectomy (Serafetinides, 1965), suggesting that either the epilepsy itself or epileptiform discharges were the cause of the aggression. However, no recent convincing studies confirming these original results were found. In particular, the recent paper by Andresen et al. (2014) did not appear to confirm the resolution of aggression with either right or left temporal lobectomy in children or teenagers.

Fohlen et al. (2004) have described "behavioural seizures" arising from the frontal lobe, revealed with invasive EEG monitoring. Frontal lobe discharges can result in disinhibited behaviour. These can be treated either with medication or surgery. Removal of the frontal lobe focus that is the source of the epileptiform discharges can improve behaviour remarkably, in some subjects, in the personal experience of the authors (unpublished work), and consistent with the work of Andresen et al. (2014). They reported marked behavioural improvements in children and teenagers undergoing frontal lobe resections, although it should be noted that their paper does not specifically document frequent frontal lobe discharges before the surgery.

The so-called benign epilepsy with centrotemporal (Rolandic) spikes was previously considered to be benign both from the point view of the prognosis for the epilepsy and in terms of any cognitive or behavioural effects. However, over recent years, data has shown that this condition can be associated with a number of adverse cognitive effects and can also be associated with attention deficit hyperactivity disorder (ADHD) (Holtmann et al., 2003) (*Behavioural and psychiatric disorders associated with childhood epilepsy syndromes*, p. XX-XX). In such circumstances, treatment of the epilepsy, together with EEG monitoring to check whether the epileptiform discharges and any apparently associated cognitive/behavioural problems have resolved, would appear to be warranted. There is still limited data to confirm this.

An extreme example of focal discharges is that of hemispheric epileptiform discharges. A cerebral hemisphere can be the source of such epileptiform discharges from a number of different causes, including Rasmussen encephalitis, cortical malformations or vascular lesions. Pharmacotherapy with antiepileptic medication is typically ineffective. Hemispherectomy, involving either the anatomical removal or the disconnection of the affected hemisphere can render the subject free from both the seizures and the behavioural disturbance. Several reviews, incorporating many patients, have concluded this in teenagers and in adults (Goodman, 1986; Lindsay et al., 1987), although the data have been open to question. The overall outcome depends very much on pre-surgical abilities and ongoing or recurrent post-surgical seizures (Moosa et al., 2013) (*Behavioural effects of epilepsy surgery*, p. XX-XX).

Absence seizures

In the past, absence seizures were said to have occurred in children that had no accompanying cognitive or behavioural problems but more recent studies have indicated a high rate of psychiatric disorder, including attention problems, anxiety, depression and somatic complaints (Caplan et al., 2008; Vega et al., 2011).

In addition, in some children, the absence seizures can be very frequent. Prolonged monitoring over 24 hours has shown that occasionally children can have not only hundreds but thousands of spike-wave episodes per day (Besag, 2011). In the most extreme case, the child may be drifting in and out of nonconvulsive status epilepticus. Although this has not been well documented in the literature, research by the current authors has shown that children who are having such frequent absence seizures can have major problems with cognition and behaviour. It is not surprising that frequent absence seizures may present with a condition that mimics attention deficit hyperactivity disorder, with the important difference that the features of attention deficit are not necessarily pervasive over time: the onset can be relatively sudden and the time course can be variable. However, the most important difference is that the features of ADHD in this situation are usually treatable with antiepileptic medication; if the cause is frequent absence seizures, stimulant medication will probably not be required. The situation is, however, complex because ADHD is, in any case, common in children with epilepsy, occurring in around 30% (Hermann et al., 2007), and a large proportion of these children respond to stimulant medication. If frequent absence seizures are present or if frequent epileptiform discharges are detected, then the first-line treatment should be with antiepileptic medication. However, those children with residual features of ADHD often respond well to stimulant medication. Contrary to past concerns, examination of the evidence indicates that there is no contraindication to prescribing stimulant medication in children with epilepsy (*Epilepsy and ADHD*, p. XX-XX).

■ Treatment of the epilepsy leading to behavioural or psychiatric disturbance

Phenobarbital, the benzodiazepines and sometimes vigabatrin can result in gross behavioural disturbance, especially in younger children (*When should pharmacotherapy for behavioural/psychiatric disorders in children with epilepsy be prescribed?*, p. XX-XX). An ADHD-like pattern of behaviour can emerge, which is reversible on discontinuing the medication. However, it should be noted that discontinuing phenobarbital or benzodiazepine drugs after prolonged use can result in withdrawal seizures, implying that, if these drugs have been taken for several months or years, they should be decreased slowly. With regard to the exact rate at which these drugs can safely be withdrawn, there are no clear guidelines based on good data. In practice, the withdrawal is usually planned to take place over weeks or months, with close monitoring for seizure exacerbations. If the seizure control deteriorates during the drug withdrawal, it may be necessary to reverse the most recent decrease, wait for a few weeks and then withdraw the medication even more slowly. Alternatively, it may be advisable to review any concomitant antiepileptic medication to achieve more stable control.

Vigabatrin and topiramate can precipitate psychosis in both adults and teenagers (Besag, 2001). The work of Mula et al. (2003) in adults has indicated that starting at a low dose and escalating slowly is likely to minimise this adverse effect. Patients with a personal or family history of psychosis should be monitored particularly carefully. There is also evidence that levetiracetam can precipitate psychosis in young people (Kossoff et al., 2001; Halma et al., 2014).

Vigabatrin and topiramate (Besag, 2001) have also been associated with depression in studies on adults but there seems to be a lack of published data in teenagers and children.

Reports on the behavioural adverse effects of gabapentin in children are conflicting. Some publications suggests that gabapentin can be associated with a deterioration of behaviour, particularly in children with pre-existing psychiatric disorders, such as ADHD (Khurana et al., 1996; Lee et al., 1996), whereas another study (Besag, 1996) found no such deterioration and behaviour in a group of teenagers with epilepsy, most of whom also had intellectual disability.

With regard to antiepileptic treatments other than medication, adult data indicate that vagus nerve stimulation can have positive effects on psychiatric symptoms, particularly depression (Klinkenberg et al., 2012). There is limited data on psychotropic effects of vagus nerve stimulation in children and teenagers (Hallböök et al., 2005).

Epilepsy neurosurgery can result either in an improvement or deterioration in behaviour. The results for resective surgery are conflicting. As already stated, hemispherectomy appears to be associated with a marked improvement in behaviour, in at least some cases, although firm evidence remains elusive (*Behavioural effects of epilepsy surgery*, p. XX-XX).

Reactions to the epilepsy

Limitations, for example the need for supervision when taking a bath, prohibition from climbing trees and other restrictions can, understandably, lead to negative reactions from the child. Pharmacotherapy for any behavioural disturbance resulting from this cause would be entirely inappropriate. Sensitive management with careful explanation of why the limitations have been imposed, with emphasis on what the child can still do, despite the epilepsy, are appropriate strategies.

Associated brain damage/dysfunction

The epidemiological work of Sillanpää (1992) indicated that 31% of children with epilepsy in a region of Finland had intellectual disability (IQ < 70). The high rate of learning problems has been confirmed in more recent studies (Reilly et al., 2014). The general trend is that as the IQ decreases, behavioural problems increase. There are many possible reasons for the intellectual disability that occurs in a large proportion of children with epilepsy. In some cases the same underlying brain condition causes both the epilepsy and intellectual disability. In a minority of cases prolonged status epilepticus can cause brain damage with accompanying intellectual disability and behavioural difficulties. In a further subgroup, traumatic brain injury can cause intellectual disability, epilepsy and behavioural problems. Each child needs to be evaluated individually. The type of behavioural disturbance can fall anywhere within a wide range, depending on the precise cause.

Pharmacotherapy can be helpful in some cases. If the clinical presentation is one of impulsivity or ADHD, stimulant medication is sometimes of benefit. If the intellectual disability is in association with autism then anxiolytic medication such as risperidone may be of benefit (Mcdougle et al., 1998).

Some children have an uneven cognitive profile. A child with disproportionately poor verbal skills may become frustrated and lash out at other people. In such circumstances, teaching the child how to use their strengths to overcome their weaknesses can be very empowering. This is not a situation in which pharmacotherapy is likely to be appropriate.

Causes that also apply to children without epilepsy

The rate of psychiatric disorder in the general childhood population is high, as demonstrated by a number of epidemiological studies, revealing rates of around 7 to 10% (Rutter et al., 1970; Davies et al., 2003; Reilly et al., 2014). Epilepsy does not protect the child against any of the disorders that might otherwise occur. However, in addition, as already stated, there is a high psychiatric comorbidity in children with epilepsy. There are several underlying reasons for this comorbidity, including a probable underlying genetic predisposition, the high rate of intellectual disability in children with epilepsy and other causes, already discussed. The key question is whether the same treatments can be used for children with epilepsy as are used in the general population of children who have psychiatric disorders. The associations between epilepsy and ADHD, autism, anxiety, depression and psychosis have been discussed in separate papers in this issue. Broadly speaking, the same medication that is used for psychiatric disorders in the general childhood population can be used for children with epilepsy, with few exceptions. Some medications, for example imipramine and clozapine, have been associated with seizure exacerbations in adults with epilepsy but even in these cases, if the dose is kept low, the probability of a serious seizure exacerbation is likely to be small (Rosenstein et al., 1993; Varma et al., 2011). However, in all cases, psychotropic medication should only be considered after careful assessment to ensure that the diagnosis is correct and that the apparent psychiatric disorder is not a direct effect of ongoing seizures/epileptiform activity, antiepileptic medication or environmental factors.

■ Conclusions

The most important step in managing the child with epilepsy and psychiatric/behavioural disorder is to carry out a very careful assessment. The specific framework suggested in this paper may act as a suitable guide for carrying out such an assessment. Before considering psychotropic medication, the possible roles of the epilepsy itself, antiepileptic medication, environmental factors and other issues should be considered carefully. If all these factors have been assessed carefully and managed appropriately, there are very few contraindications for prescribing psychotropic medication. The wise prescription of such medication can be of great benefit in appropriately selected cases.

References

Andresen EN, Ramirez MJ, Kim KH, Dorfman AB, Haut JS, Klaas PA, et al. Effects of surgical side and site on mood and behavior outcome in children with pharmacoresistant epilepsy. *Front Neurol* 2014; 5: 18.

Besag FMC. Subtle cognitive and behavioral effects of epilepsy. In: Trimble M & Schmitz B (eds.) *The Neuropsychiatry of Epilepsy*. 2nd ed. Cambridge, UK: Cambridge University Press, 2011: 39-45.

Besag FMC. Childhood Epilepsy in Relation to Mental Handicap and Behavioural Disorders. *Journal of Child Psychology & Psychiatry & Allied Disciplines* 2002a; 43(1): 103-131.

Besag FMC. When is it inappropriate to prescribe psychotropic medication? *Epilepsia* 2002b; 43 Suppl 2: 45-50.

Besag FMC. Behavioural effects of the new anticonvulsants. *Drug Safety* 2001; 24(7): 513-536.

Besag FMC. Gabapentin use with paediatric patients. *Reviews in Contemporary Pharmacotherapy* 1996; 7(5): 233-238.

Caplan R, Siddarth P, Stahl L, Lanphier E, Vona P, Gurbani S, et al. Childhood absence epilepsy: behavioral, cognitive, and linguistic comorbidities. *Epilepsia* 2008; 49(11): 1838-1846.

Davies S, Heyman I, Goodman R. A population survey of mental health problems in children with epilepsy. *Developmental Medicine & Child Neurology* 2003; 45(5): 292-295.

Devinsky O, Honigfeld G, Patin J. Clozapine-related seizures. *Neurology* 1991; 41(3): 369-371.

Fenton GW. Epilepsy and automatism. *Br J Psychiatry* 1975; Spec No 9: 429-39.

Fohlen M, Bulteau C, Jalin C, Jambaque I, Delalande O. Behavioural epileptic seizures: a clinical and intracranial EEG study in 8 children with frontal lobe epilepsy. *Neuropediatrics* 2004; 35(6): 336-345.

Goodman R. Hemispherectomy and its alternatives in the treatment of intractable epilepsy in patients with infantile hemiplegia. *Developmental Medicine & Child Neurology* 1986; 28(2): 251-258.

Gupta AK, Jeavons PM, Hughes RC, Covanis A. Aura in temporal lobe epilepsy: clinical and electroencephalographic correlation. *Journal of Neurology, Neurosurgery & Psychiatry* 1983; 46(12): 1079-1083.

Hallböök T, Lundgren J, Stjernqvist K, Blennow G, Strömblad LG, Rosén I. Vagus nerve stimulation in 15 children with therapy resistant epilepsy; its impact on cognition, quality of life, behaviour and mood. *Seizure* 2005; 14(7): 504-513.

Halma E, De Louw A, Klinkenberg S, Aldenkamp A, Ijff D, Majoie M. Behavioral side-effects of levetiracetam in children with epilepsy: a systematic review. *Seizure* 2014; 23(9): 685-91.

Hermann B, Jones J, Dabbs K, Allen CA, Sheth R, Fine J, et al. The frequency, complications and aetiology of ADHD in new onset paediatric epilepsy. *Brain* 2007; 130(Pt:12): 12-48.

Holtmann M, Becker K, Kentner-Figura B, Schmidt MH. Increased frequency of rolandic spikes in ADHD children. *Epilepsia* 2003; 44(9): 1241-1244.

Kanemoto K, Kawasaki J, Kawai I. Postictal psychosis: a comparison with acute interictal and chronic psychoses. *Epilepsia* 1996; 37(6): 551-6.

Kanner AM, Soto A, Gross-Kanner H. Prevalence and clinical characteristics of postictal psychiatric symptoms in partial epilepsy. *Neurology* 2004; 62(5): 708-13.

Kaufmann R, Goldberg-Stern H, Shuper A. Attention-deficit disorders and epilepsy in childhood: incidence, causative relations and treatment possibilities. *J Child Neurol* 2009; 24(6): 727-33.

Khurana DS, Riviello J, Helmers S, Holmes G, Anderson J, Mikati MA. Efficacy of gabapentin therapy in children with refractory partial seizures. *Journal of Pediatrics* 1996; 128(6): 829-833.

Klinkenberg S, Majoie HJ, Van Der Heijden MM, Rijkers K, Leenen L, Aldenkamp AP. Vagus nerve stimulation has a positive effect on mood in patients with refractory epilepsy. *Clinical Neurology & Neurosurgery* 2012; 114(4): 336-340.

Kossoff EH, Bergey GK, Freeman JM, Vining EP. Levetiracetam psychosis in children with epilepsy. *Epilepsia* 2001; 42(12): 1611-1613.

Lee DO, Steingard RJ, Cesena M, Helmers SL, Riviello JJ, Mikati MA. Behavioral side effects of gabapentin in children. *Epilepsia* 1996; 37(1): 87-90.

Lennox WG, Cobb S. Epilepsy: XIII. Aura in epilepsy; a statistical review of 1,359 cases. *Archives of Neurology and Psychiatry* 1933; 30(2): 374.

Lindsay J, Ounsted C, Richards P. Hemispherectomy for childhood epilepsy: a 36-year study. *Developmental Medicine & Child Neurology* 1987; 29(5): 592-600.

Mcdougle CJ, Holmes JP, Carlson DC, Pelton GH, Cohen DJ, Price LH. A double-blind, placebo-controlled study of risperidone in adults with autistic disorder and other pervasive developmental disorders. *Archives of General Psychiatry* 1998; 55(7): 633-641.

Mcintyre J, Robertson S, Norris E, Appleton R, Whitehouse WP, Phillips B, et al. Safety and efficacy of buccal midazolam versus rectal diazepam for emergency treatment of seizures in children: a randomised controlled trial. *Lancet* 2005; 366(9481): 205-210.

Moosa AN, Gupta A, Jehi L, Marashly A, Cosmo G, Lachhwani D, et al. Longitudinal seizure outcome and prognostic predictors after hemispherectomy in 170 children. *Neurology* 2013; 80(3): 253-60.

Mula M, Trimble MR, Lhatoo SD, Sander JW. Topiramate and psychiatric adverse events in patients with epilepsy. *Epilepsia* 2003; 44(5): 659-663.

Pisani F, Oteri G, Costa C, Di Raimondo G, Di Perri R. Effects of psychotropic drugs on seizure threshold. *Drug Safety* 2002; 25(2): 91-110.

Rajna P, Clemens B, Csibri E, Dobos E, Geregely A, Gottschal M, *et al*. Hungarian multicentre epidemiologic study of the warning and initial symptoms (prodrome, aura) of epileptic seizures. *Seizure* 1997; 6(5): 361-368.

Reilly C, Atkinson P, Das KB, Chin RF, Aylett SE, Burch V, *et al*. Neurobehavioral comorbidities in children with active epilepsy: a population-based study. *Pediatrics* 2014; 133(6): e1586-93.

Rosenstein DL, Nelson JC, Jacobs SC. Seizures associated with antidepressants: a review. *Journal of Clinical Psychiatry* 1993; 54(8): 289-299.

Rutter M, Graham P, Yule W. *A neuropsychiatric study in childhood*, London, Heinemann Medical, 1970.

Scheffer IE, Bhatia KP, Lopes-Cendes I, Fish DR, Marsden CD, Andermann E, *et al*. Autosomal dominant nocturnal frontal lobe epilepsy. A distinctive clinical disorder. *Brain* 1995; 118 (Pt 1): 61-73.

Scott RC, Besag FMC, Neville BGR. Buccal midazolam and rectal diazepam for treatment of prolonged seizures in childhood and adolescence: A randomised trial. *Lancet* 1999; 353(9153): 623-626.

Serafetinides EA. Aggressiveness in Temporal Lobe Epileptics and Its Relation to Cerebral Dysfunction and Environmental Factors. *Epilepsia* 1965; 6: 33-42.

Sillanpää M. Epilepsy in children: prevalence, disability, and handicap. *Epilepsia* 1992; 33(3): 444-449.

Treiman DM. Epilepsy and violence: medical and legal issues. *Epilepsia* 1986; 27(Suppl 2): S77-S104.

Varma S, Bishara D, Besag FMC, Taylor D. Clozapine-related EEG changes and seizures: dose and plasma-level relationships. *Ther Adv Psychopharmacol* 2011; 1(2): 47-66.

Vega C, Guo J, Killory B, Danielson N, Vestal M, Berman R, *et al*. Symptoms of anxiety and depression in childhood absence epilepsy. *Epilepsia* 2011; 52(8): e70-4.

Wolf SM, Forsythe A. Behavior disturbance, phenobarbital, and febrile seizures. *Pediatrics* 1978; 61(5): 728-31.

Table 1. Recommended pharmacotherapy for psychiatric/behavioural disorders

Situation/Issue	Pharmacotherapy	Comments
Prodrome	No specific treatment. It is anticipated that complete seizure control should also control prodrome.	The possibility that incomplete antiepileptic treatment could result in more prominent prodromes has been suggested but has not been established
Aura	Intermittent bouts of very frequent auras can be treated with single doses or brief courses of an oral benzodiazepine such as clobazam	There is lack of published data to support this strategy, which appears to be effective in practice
Automatism	Complete seizure control should also control seizure-related automatisms.	Automatisms are not always recognised as such; the importance of taking a meticulous history cannot be over-emphasised.
Post-ictal psychosis	Postictal psychosis may be self-limiting but if it is causing distress or associated with risk, treatment with antipsychotic medication is indicated.	Risk of seizure exacerbation with antipsychotic medication is relatively low and related to dose. Clozapine can precipitate seizures; however, again the effect is dose-related.
Interictal psychoses	May require longer-term treatment with antipsychotic medication.	(As above.) Risk of seizure exacerbation with antipsychotic medication is relatively low and probably related to dose. Clozapine can precipitate seizures; however, again the effect is dose-related.
Focal epileptiform discharges	Treatment with antiepileptic medication might be of benefit but surgical treatment in suitably-selected cases is definitive	Some evidence for significant behavioural improvement after left temporal lobectomy or frontal lobe resection for frequent focal discharges. Anatomical or functional hemispherectomy can be associated both with seizure freedom and behavioural improvement
Absence seizures	Treat with standard anti-absence AEDs	Lamotrigine is favoured because of positive psychotropic effects, although ethosuximide is more effective. Avoid valproate in females of child-bearing potential
ADHD	Assess carefully (see text) but do not withhold standard ADHD medication such as methylphenidate, dexamfetamine, atomoxetine or clonidine if indicated	Risk of seizure exacerbation with ADHD treatment such as methylphenidate, dexamfetamine, atomoxetine or clonidine appears to be very low
Anxiety associated with autism spectrum disorder	Low-dose risperidone can be highly effective. Typically commence at 0.25 mg once or twice daily, escalating every 3 to 7 days until favourable response or until plateau reached, keeping to minimum effective dose, typically around 0.5 mg twice daily. Alternatives are aripiprazole or olanzapine	Low-dose antipsychotic medication is unlikely to cause seizure exacerbations. Weight gain can occur with all three antipsychotics, tending to be greatest with olanzapine and least with aripiprazole.

Generalised anxiety	Assess carefully and ensure that epilepsy-related causes, for example auras, are managed appropriately. If selective serotonin reuptake inhibitors are indicated, they should not be withheld	Seizure exacerbations are unlikely to occur with selective serotonin reuptake inhibitors, which might even raise the seizure threshold
Depression	If lifestyle limitations resulting from the epilepsy are the cause of low mood, antidepressant medication is unlikely to be of benefit. Talking therapy is generally favoured as first-line treatment in children and teenagers but selective serotonin reuptake inhibitors should not be withheld, if indicated.	As above – seizure exacerbations are unlikely to occur with selective serotonin reuptake inhibitors, which might even raise the seizure threshold

IMPRIM'VERT®

Achevé d'imprimer par 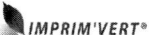 Corlet, Imprimeur, S.A.
14110 Condé-sur-Noireau
N° d'Imprimeur : 182927 - Dépôt légal : juillet 2016
Imprimé en France